AUTISM SPECTRUM DISORDER:

PRACTICAL HANDBOOK FOR

CAREGIVERS
IN SELF-CARE

What Caregivers Need to Know in
Parenting a Happy and Strong ASD Child?
Take Care of Yourself First.
Your Autistic Child Comes Next.

EUNICE CHURCHILL

TABLE OF CONTENTS

INTRODUCTION

Nowadays, most self-care guides and resources out there encourage people to adopt a "well-balanced routine." We read about how daily exercise, good food habits, meditation, healthy distractions, and open communication can help us become the happiest and most productive version of ourselves. When it comes to raising and/or caring for individuals with autism, finding that balance is a much trickier endeavor. It can be difficult to prioritize self-care when most of your life revolves around fulfilling that individual's special needs. Devoting your time and energy to care for someone else is very admirable, but it can also burn you out if you're not careful.

This book is designed specifically to help empower ASD caregivers. Whether you're a parent, relative, friend, teacher, or therapist, you'll find techniques and tools to better navigate the challenges that come with looking after an autistic child. The focus of this book comes down to one essential precept: Enabling yourself to be and feel better about your duties will allow you to better care for others in return. While it may sound easier said than done, learning how to prioritize your own well-being, mentally and emotionally, can yield extraordinarily positive results. It may even help you rekindle a strong sense of purpose.

As we all know, neglecting our own needs can be quite detrimental to our well-being. That's why this comprehensive guide provides a roadmap to help you become more resilient as an ASD caregiver. Chapter after chapter, you'll grow your knowledge of autism, its main challenges, and obstacles, how to seek support, and the importance of self-care rituals. It will teach you many essential skills for managing your own mental health in the long run.

It's been established that the early years are critical for any person's cognitive and neural development. As it happens, children with ASD have special needs that aren't always easy to accommodate. Because they don't develop as effortlessly as their peers, this often puts a great deal of pressure and stress on their caregivers, which takes a great emotional toll on them and their quality of life. In time, this can hinder a person's ability to deliver effective and compassionate care. Fortunately, there are several proven ways to strike a healthy balance and remind yourself of how proud you are to be someone else's devoted caregiver.

Ultimately, looking after an individual with autism is a very demanding responsibility. We don't always have the right reflexes, and our minds are rarely at ease when taking care of them. Hopefully, what you're about to read will offer a fresh perspective to help you approach your caregiving duties with renewed faith and confidence. Without further ado, let's discover how you can make a difference in the lives of those who need you by implementing changes in your own life.

CHAPTER ONE

WHAT IT MEANS TO BE A CAREGIVER FOR INDIVIDUALS WITH AUTISM SPECTRUM DISORDER

Although Autism Spectrum Disorder (ASD) is usually diagnosed during the developmental stages of childhood, individuals can sometimes reach adulthood before a proper assessment takes place. In cases where ASD affects an individual's ability to care for themselves, they will require a caregiver for the rest of their life. This means that the role of caregiver can be parents, siblings, other family members, friends, or professional healthcare workers. This is a long-term commitment undertaken by caregivers, and it's often a full-time job. Anyone who is going to be taking on a caregiver role, or those already acting as caregivers for individuals with ASD, need to be aware of what this responsibility actually means before they agree to become a caregiver.

What Is Autism Spectrum Disorder?

Autism Spectrum Disorder (ASD) is a neurological and developmental disorder that affects a person's ability to communicate, interact with others, and causes repetitive behaviors. It can pose considerable challenges in regard to behavior, learning, communication, and sociability, especially in children of young age. ASD is a "spectrum" because it affects people in different ways and to different degrees. Those with a mild case of ASD will generally grow up and live with relative autonomy, but severe cases will require far more daily care, monitoring, and emotional support to thrive. Some people with ASD are nonverbal and need a significant amount of assistance in all aspects of their life.

There is no one-size-fits-all profile for someone who has ASD, but there are a handful of common symptoms used when making a diagnosis. These can include difficulty with eye contact and social interaction, repetitive speech or movements, high levels of anxiety, and sensory processing issues. People with ASD often have difficulty understanding the emotions of others, which can make social interactions very challenging. People with ASD can also excel at a particular subject or activity, like math or playing an instrument. In some cases, early intervention and therapy can help lessen the symptoms of ASD, but there is no cure for the disorder. Despite the challenges associated with ASD, many people with the disorder go on to lead happy and successful lives.

Why Caregivers are Important to Individuals with ASD

Someone with ASD may have difficulty with communication and social interaction. This can make it hard to form relationships and connect with others. Fortunately, there are people who can help you manage your autism and navigate the world. These people are called caregivers, and they play an important role in their life.

Caregivers provide their charges with support and assistance with their daily activities. They can aid with things like communication, grooming, and eating. They can also help you engage in activities that are enjoyable and stimulating. In addition, caregivers can provide them with emotional support. They can be a listening ear when an individual with ASD needs to talk and a shoulder to cry on when feeling down. Caregivers are an important part of a support system. They can help their charges manage autism and help them live a full and happy life.

Who Can Be a Caretaker?

- Parents
- Family members
- Professional Healthcare Workers

- Therapists
- Teachers

Caring for a Child with ASD

A child with ASD is a special needs child who requires more care and attention than a neurotypical child. Their brains process and learn information differently than other children's. Their physical body may develop normally, but their intellect is delayed. How you treat the child as they grow will contribute to their ability to psychologically cope with the challenges they will encounter throughout their lives, as well as their confidence in themselves as a person. By emphasizing that ASD doesn't need to define them, you can help your child understand that they can become whatever kind of person they desire.

Parents can't wait to watch their children develop independence as they start to handle things on their own, but you'll need to put in a lot of effort to see this through. It would be a mistake to view ASD as something needing to be "cured." Many parents try various treatments on their children, hoping to obtain permanent recovery, which is a mirage. The best you can do is learn to manage the condition properly. Caring for a child is determining how you assist them in developing self-confidence, independence, and trust in you, good relationships with others, being a happy child, and having a healthy mind, body, and spirit. Since ASD is incurable, it does not preclude you from managing the situation and raising an autonomous, happy child.

Be Involved in Your Child's Treatment

Be sure to voice any concerns or ask questions about your child's treatment. You must understand the treatment goals and how they will be achieved.

You can learn more about ASD and how to support your child by attending parent training programs. Local autism organizations or universities often offer these programs.

Regularly follow up with your child's treatment team and service providers to ensure your child is progressing and receiving the best possible care.

Promote Social Skills

You can help your child develop social skills by modeling appropriate behavior and providing opportunities for practice. Playdates with other children are a great way for your child to practice social skills. You can also enroll them in social skills groups or therapy programs.

Encourage Language Development

Help your child develop language skills by talking to them often, reading books, and singing songs. It is important to use words that your child can understand and provide simple explanations. Also, help your child develop language skills by enrolling them in speech therapy programs.

It is important to note that many children with ASD struggle with verbal communication. However, they are able to communicate in other ways, such as through sign language, picture boards, or apps.

Enhance Learning Opportunities

Help your child to learn by providing opportunities for practice and encouraging their interests. Many children with ASD excel in visual learning, so help your child learn using flashcards, picture books, and videos. Also, make sure to provide opportunities for hands-on learning, including puzzles, building blocks, and drawing.

Teach Your Child New Skills

Help your child learn new skills by breaking down tasks into small steps and teaching them one step at a time. Be sure to praise your child for their successes and be patient with them when they make mistakes.

Promote Physical Activity

Physical activity is important for all children, including those with ASD. It improves motor skills, promotes social interaction, and reduces stress.

You can help your child be active by enrolling them in sports programs without physical contact or taking them for walks or bike rides together.

Reduce Stress

Reduce your child's stress by maintaining a routine, providing clear explanations, and avoiding overwhelming situations. You can achieve this by including regular exercise, eating a healthy diet, and getting enough sleep in your daily routine.

Develop Routines

Routines reduce stress and provide a sense of security for children with ASD. You can develop routines by setting regular times for meals, sleep, and activities. It is also important to be consistent with rules and expectations.

It is proven that children with ASD thrive when their environment is predictable. So, developing routines makes your child's world more predictable and less stressful.

Be Patient

It is important to be patient when communicating with your child and avoid rushing them. Being patient with them reduces stress and promotes effective communication.

Also, it is essential to be patient when your child engages in repetitive behaviors. These behaviors are often a way for your child to cope with stress.

Be a Good Role Model

You can help your child develop social skills by being a good role model. Demonstrate appropriate social skills, and be sure to praise your child when they use these skills. By being a good role model, you help your child to learn and practice appropriate social behavior.

Encourage Your Child's Interests

Encourage your child's interests and help them to pursue their passions. This will help your child feel good about themselves and give them a sense of purpose.

It's vital to provide opportunities for your child to socialize with others who share their interests; this helps your child make friends and feel more connected to the community.

Be Your Child's Biggest Advocate

The wonderful thing about understanding everything there is to know about autism and paying attention to your child's specific requirements is that it helps you determine every detail of your child's feelings and needs. You will understand what makes your child happy or unhappy, what they find difficult and what brings them joy, and what makes the child calm or worried. It will help you find strategies to avoid disruptive behaviors from occurring or the best approach to resolve them. Allow your child to have less of what scares or stresses them and more of what makes them excited and relaxed.

Be sure to advocate for your child's rights and needs, including working with schools and service providers to ensure that your child receives the best possible education and services. Advocate for your child by staying informed about ASD and sharing information with family and friends.

Be There for Them

The most important thing you can do for your child is to be present and involved in their life, including spending time together, discussing their day, and listening to their concerns.

Moreover, providing emotional support and being a source of strength during difficult times is crucial for your child. By being there for your child, you can help them to feel loved and supported.

Reach Out for Support

Caring for children with special needs is a challenge and should never be faced alone if possible. Whenever you feel stressed or overwhelmed, reach out to your family and friends for support. A simple conversation about your difficulties can sometimes be sufficient to put them in perspective and help you overcome them. There are also many resources available for parents of children with ASD. These resources provide information, advice, and emotional support.

Remember: you are not alone in this journey. There are people who care about you and your child, and are more than willing to help. A community of parents, professionals, and advocates is always available to support you. Working with this community will provide the best possible outcome for children with ASD. Let's make an inclusive world for all where children with special needs are celebrated and not merely tolerated.

When friends and family are not an option, parents of special needs children can find support in local support groups and online chat groups. Various mental health apps are available to let you vent or talk through your problems. You can cope better with your struggles if you share them with others going through the same thing. Some of the most valuable advice is provided by those who have previously experienced it.

Caring for Adults with ASD

While all children require caregivers, regardless of the severity of their ASD, any adults who need one tend to be on the more extreme end of the spectrum. An adult with ASD is going to have different needs and routines than a child, as they are well past the developmental period in their lives. However, it can be just as demanding on a caregiver's time and energy—sometimes even more so. Depending on the level of communication abilities an adult with ASD is at, caregivers may need to assist them with things like speech therapy and behavioral management.

An adult with ASD may never reach a psychological and emotional maturity beyond that of a child, but their bodies will continue to age physically. This means that they will experience all the problems that accompany aging, but struggle with understanding why these changes are happening and how to deal with it. Maintaining a consistent schedule and continuity in their environment is immensely important to help manage an adult with ASD. As they develop different needs over time, slowly tweaking their routines in incremental ways can often be the best way to help meet those requirements.

Keep Calm and Be Empathetic

Adults with ASD are dealing with a lot of issues, including difficulty regulating their feelings and emotions, despite having reached physical maturity. Conversations can quickly turn frustrating, not just for you, but for them as well. Being patient and understanding is key, and you should never try to rush them, as it will only serve to cause more stress. When people with ASD become overwhelmed, that's when they begin to shut down and retreat to the types of repetitive behaviors that children do, such as hitting a wall over and over, or shouting, "No! No! No!"

Navigating the problems of ASD is something a caregiver will have to learn to do in conjunction with their charge. Sensory overload is often something that people with ASD will retain their entire lives, so you have to keep a close watch on anything that might trigger them. Try to stay calm, no matter what else is happening at the moment. Those with ASD might have an outburst, but if you show them that there's nothing wrong by using a comforting tone of voice and not expressing anger, it's more likely that they'll pick up on that and calm down, too.

Personal Space

It can be hard to give a person whose welfare is your responsibility their space, but just like you, adults with ASD need to have some time to themselves. While their development may not have progressed to that of a neurotypical adult, they can still have the desire to do something on their own, like play a game or practice an instrument. If the person you're caring for has proven they can handle being alone for an hour or so, you can both use the opportunity to practice some self-care.

Another thing to remember is that many individuals with ASD aren't always comfortable with typical conventions of social interaction. Trying to maintain eye contact with others might make them feel awkward, and while there are times where gently urging them to look someone in the eyes while speaking is a good thing, you have to learn to pick up on the signs that you should back off. Affection and touching is something else that can be uncomfortable for someone with ASD, so don't ever try to force intimacy on them, even if they're family.

The Effects of Aging

Unfortunately, people with ASD are at a higher risk of health complications as they transition from middle age to their senior years. This is because they often can't comprehend what's happening to their bodies, and they may not be able to effectively communicate when something is wrong. It can be a very traumatic experience, and even adults with ASD who were mostly self-sufficient can start requiring a caregiver full-time. Then you have to consider all the regular issues that come with aging, such as Alzheimer's Disease or Dementia.

Caring for an elderly individual with ASD can be an incredibly difficult challenge. You have to keep a very close watch on their health, especially tracking any changes in their behavior or demeanor that could indicate a potential problem, since they may not be able to alert you about it. Confusion over their thoughts and emotions can get worse, and as their ability to communicate deteriorates, there is greater risk of an undiagnosed ailment causing serious damage to their health before it's addressed.

CHAPTER TWO

THE IMPORTANCE OF SELF-CARE FOR CAREGIVERS

Almost 90 million people in the EU are classed as the main caregiver of children under the age of 15. But how many of these people also take care of themselves? Caring for others sometimes leaves little time for self-care, which is just as important. Being a caregiver for anyone can place a strain on your physical, emotional, and mental health. Caring for someone with autism is even more demanding and challenging. You often find yourself preoccupied with their demands, and you could underestimate the impact this has on you and those around you.

Failure to respond to your own self-care requirements can have a long-term detrimental influence on your physical, emotional, and mental health. If your well-being suffers, your ability to provide proper care can suffer as well. Practicing self-care not only helps you to recharge and feel more capable of meeting the demands of your caregiving role, but helps you to be the best caregiver possible. When you're well-rested and have the energy to care for your loved one, you'll handle difficult situations more effectively.

In addition, self-care helps reduce stress and anxiety. Taking time for yourself allows you to recharge and return to your role as a caregiver with a fresh perspective. Furthermore, self-care will improve your physical health. When you're feeling physically well, you are better equipped to handle the challenges of caregiving. Make sure to schedule some time for yourself every day, even if it's just a few minutes. Your loved one with autism will benefit from a happier, healthier caregiver.

It Takes a Lot of Effort to Care for Others

Caregivers of people with ASD are usually working full-time in their role. They often need to be available all day and overnight to deal with any problems that might occur. This means you will be required to:

- Possess the stamina and ability to work continuously for long periods
- Ability to handle stress well
- Accept a limited social life
- Be industrious and persevering
- Work alone, without recognition or praise in isolation
- Operate and inside the medical and health

professional field

- Earn a low income or none at all

The above are only a few issues caretakers face, and it is clear this is a selfless task that deserves respect. Caregivers need care and support to be physically and mentally strong to continue providing care. However, parents must avoid allowing parenting to consume them. Parents must understand how fatigue affects their health and develop a self-care plan to combat it.

Insufficient support can make caring for a child with special needs an overwhelming full-time job. Caregiver burnout has a detrimental effect on all involved if parents do not receive enough help or have the appropriate tips to stay above water.

What is Self-Care?

Self-care is the practice of proactively taking action to protect or improve your health and preserve or increase your happiness and well-being. This means taking some time out of your day to do things that offer relief from stress and fortifying your mental, emotional, and physical health. The definition of self-care is found in the term itself - caring for oneself. Self-care includes prioritizing your physical, mental, and emotional well-being.

Those who have difficulty letting go must understand that taking steps to care for themselves does not equate to selfishness or pleasure-seeking. Self-care merely means considering how being healthy will benefit those involved in the caring process.

While your charges rely on you to provide care for them, you don't have a caregiver of your own, so you must take on the responsibility to care for yourself. This isn't selfish, although it might feel that way when the individual with ASD you're taking care of needs so much attention. Self-care isn't about prioritizing your health over theirs any more than you should prioritize their health over yours. There is a balance that must be struck between the two in order to maximize the benefits for all parties involved.

There isn't a single, "best" method to go about practicing self-care. It depends on many different variables, the main one being your threshold for stress and anxiety. How often you need to take the time to engage in a bit of self-care throughout the day will be determined by when ignoring your own needs will start to boil over and cause an impairment to your ability to provide care for others. If you find yourself reaching your "breaking point," it's a sign that you've gone too long without taking care of your own needs. Ideally, during the course of your time as a caregiver, you'll figure out how to recognize the warnings that you are beginning to become overstressed and take steps to alleviate the problem before it becomes detrimental to your caretaking capabilities.

Benefits of Practicing Self-Care

Physical and emotional exhaustion makes everyone less capable of handling the stresses life throws our way. When we are at our mental and physical best, we feel empowered and more prepared to face life's challenges. Pampering yourself with a mud face mask, a warm bubble bath, or other activities recharges the mind, body, and soul. There are many advantages to benefit your life if you take the necessary steps to care for yourself. By addressing the risks of neglecting self-care, you can avoid creating additional challenges that are easily avoidable.

Makes You a Better Caregiver

Those who neglect their own needs and do not nurture themselves risk experiencing resentment, depression, and low self-esteem. As discussed above, people who spend all their time taking care of others are more likely to suffer emotional burnout. This phenomenon is difficult to alleviate when long-term care is the norm. Regular and consistent self-care activities will help you become a better caregiver.

Improves Your Mental Health

It is essential that everyone spends some time alone now and then, whether they are caregivers or not. This is true for both introverts and extroverts. You need the opportunity to reflect on your life, goals, and worries. Spending time alone is critical for personal development and growth, which is something you should always be striving toward. Keeping yourself mentally healthy helps you think clearly and make better decisions, which are two things that are incredibly important when serving as a caregiver.

Improves Your Physical Health

Maintaining a healthy body can boost your energy and self-esteem. Remaining in good physical shape can make your responsibilities much easier, since you won't get tired out as quickly when carrying out the tasks expected of you. Being in poor health can make you irritable and quick to snap at others, which can cause even more problems when caring for people with ASD than it does with others in your life.

Improves Your Emotional Health

Emotional health isn't discussed nearly as often as physical or mental health, but that doesn't mean it's any less important to your well-being. When you are self-aware, taking the time to look inward, you remind yourself how important you are. Emotional maturity is one of the ways people prevent themselves from allowing their feelings to dictate their behavior. Caregiving can be a thankless job, and it feels awful when those being cared for take you for granted. But practicing self-care can help you recognize that there isn't a need for someone to thank you, because you know you are doing the right thing.

CHAPTER THREE

CHALLENGES FACED BY CAREGIVERS

As the parent or caregiver of an individual with ASD, you know that each day comes with its own set of challenges while providing around-the-clock care. This includes feeding, bathing, and dressing the person for whom you're caring. You may also need to help them with toileting and other basic daily tasks. They may also require assistance with communication, social interaction, and behavioral issues.

From meltdowns and tantrums to poor social skills and sensory issues, autism can present itself with a wide range of difficulties. While every person is unique, there are some common challenges that many parents and caregivers will face. Understanding the problems you will encounter can make it easier to find solutions for them, as you can analyze the situation and strategize ways to solve them while using a calm, logical mind.

Being a parent is challenging enough as it is, yet the demands of parenting a special needs child sometimes make it far more exhausting. Almost every aspect of parenting is more challenging, including helping with homework and providing for the physical and emotional needs of the child. It can be very taxing on a parent. Caring for an adult is equally challenging, but often in different ways. Recognizing the additional strain that comes with caring for someone with special needs is important.

You aren't a bad person for simply recognizing how tough being a caregiver can be. Even if you find yourself wishing you were in a different situation, what matters is your actions and how you choose to deal with your problems. Give yourself credit for everything you do as a parent or caregiver. It will help you deal with emotional and physical challenges, as you won't constantly feel guilty about needing a break every once in a while.

Communication

One of the biggest challenges faced by parents and caregivers is communication. Those with ASD often have trouble communicating their wants and needs, which can lead to frustration for you and your charge. Sometimes it feels like you must constantly guess what they're trying to tell you. However, there are ways to help them communicate more effectively, like using picture cards or sign language to help them express themselves.

Another common challenge facing parents and caregivers

is behavioral issues. Many people with ASD have difficulty regulating their emotions, resulting in outbursts or meltdowns. While it is important to help them manage their emotions, when necessary, it is also important to be understanding and patient. Remember, individuals with ASD often cannot help their behavior, and punishment will not fix the problem. Instead, be patient with them and help them learn better ways to express themselves.

Meltdowns and Tantrums

Meltdowns and tantrums are extremely common problems you'll have to deal with, especially in children. When a child with ASD becomes overwhelmed or frustrated, they can express it through crying, yelling, or lashing out physically. It isn't always easy to deal with, especially in public places. It's crucial to remember that these outbursts are not intentional—your child is merely struggling to communicate their needs. You can help your child through these tough moments with patience and understanding.

Adults with ASD may also be prone to meltdowns and becoming physically violent. In their case, it can pose a much more serious risk to the caretaker, as most adults are larger and stronger than children. It's important to be aware of these potential issues before agreeing to become a caretaker for an adult with ASD. Behavioral problems like this won't necessarily only happen when the individual becomes agitated, the way most neurotypical people will have a period of anger that builds up to physical violence. Sudden lashing out can occur even if the individual appears to be calm, so it's essential you understand this and are capable of reacting and safely defusing the situation at any moment.

Sensory Overload

Sensory issues are another common problem. Many individuals with ASD have difficulty processing and responding to information from their senses. Overstimulation can occur with any of their senses, but generally will happen with sounds, tastes, and touch. Even something as seemingly-innocuous as the tag on the inside collar of a t-shirt may trigger a sensory overload. Figuring out what types of things will cause discomfort or irritability in your charge will be essential in helping you develop a plan of care for them.

Issues with sensory overload can result in a range of behaviors, from ignoring people or objects to becoming overwhelmed easily by loud noises or the flavor and texture of certain foods. As a parent or caregiver, you want to avoid pushing a person with ASD into something that will cause them stress. Helping them cope with their sensory challenges can make their life and your own happier and healthier. You just need patience and understanding.

Time Management

The demands of caring for someone with ASD are usually around-the-clock. In addition to providing physical care, caregivers often act as advocates, educators, and therapists. They provide emotional support to family members struggling to cope with a diagnosis. This means a caretaker may spend what little time they have outside of physically caring for their charge dealing with these tertiary matters. The constant demands can lead to anxiety, depression, and isolation.

One feature of ASD is a fixation on routines. Even slight variations to the individual's typical daily routine can trigger a negative emotional response. It's important that caregivers have strong organizational skills, and taking time to prepare a schedule each day for your charge can be beneficial to ensuring you manage your time effectively. This will naturally be more difficult early on, until you start to get a sense for what routines offer the best results. Once a routine is proven to work, making sure you stick with it can aid you in avoiding other problems from cropping up.

Financial Pressure

When it comes to raising a child or caring for a family member with ASD, the financial strain can be immense. Professional caregivers will at least receive compensation for their work, but parents and family members must rely on other sources of income if they spend the majority of their time caring for someone with ASD. In a two parent household, this usually means only one parent serving as the breadwinner, as parenting a child with ASD is also a full time job. Single parents often have no choice but to hire a professional caregiver, especially if they don't have any reliable family members willing to take on the role. Professional caregivers can be expensive, and that's on top of all the regular financial responsibilities parents must consider when raising a child.

Obsessive Tendencies

One feature of ASD that is fairly consistent across the entire spectrum is a tendency toward obsessive-compulsive behavior. This manifests in many different ways, the most obvious often being a fixation on a particular piece of media or fictional character. Individuals with ASD will find something they enjoy, and then proceed to spend nearly all their time wanting to do things related to their obsession. The video game character "Sonic the Hedgehog" is a popular favorite of children with ASD, possibly because the bright colors and rapid-fire movements in Sonic games, movies, and TV shows is something that attracts them.

Obsessive tendencies can also result in a proficiency or mastery in certain subjects or activities. There are many cases where a person with ASD will pick up a musical instrument and become extremely skilled at it. Others display an almost innate understanding of a subject that has immutable rules, like mathematics. This isn't necessarily a problem, but individuals with ASD may focus so much on this one aspect of their life that they neglect all others. It's important to nurture their talents, but it's equally beneficial to encourage them to try other things and get new experiences, especially with socialization. Just like with other children, those with ASD will have a more solid foundation for later in life if they develop a well-rounded personality early on.

Behavioral Issues

Behavioral issues in people with ASD, particularly defiance or refusal to do something when asked, can be one of the biggest challenges faced by a caregiver. When the individual is uncomfortable or doesn't want to do something, it can be very difficult to discipline them, as even threats of punishment may not be enough to force compliance. This is extremely frustrating for parents and caregivers, and there isn't always a foolproof method of dealing with such behavior. One thing you must have in abundance as a caregiver is patience.

Some individuals with ASD react to change or unexpected situations by lashing out. They may stubbornly refuse to do something, or refuse to accept that they aren't allowed to do something. It's important to remember that yelling at them or speaking to them harshly isn't likely to result in a positive outcome. You can certainly be firm, but remaining calm and using an even, but authoritative voice will work better than shouting or threats of punishment. Sometimes, a person with ASD may exhibit negative behavior because they don't understand why they can or can't do something. Explaining your reasoning in a clear and concise manner may help them process why certain actions have consequences, or why they need to comply with your rules.

Caregiver Burnout

If you feel you're constantly running on empty, you're not alone. There will come a point as a caregiver where you feel overwhelmed by your responsibilities. Individuals with special needs require a lot of attention, which can be an emotionally and physically draining experience. Be mindful of the stress caregivers face daily, and take steps to manage it and avoid burnout. Needing to provide constant care for your charge isn't going to change, but you can change how you manage your time when providing this care.

What Is Caregiver Burnout?

Caregiver burnout occurs when a person is physically, emotionally, and mentally exhausted from managing the wants and needs of an individual with ASD. For example, when caregivers lack social or professional help, or if they take on more than they should, financially or emotionally, a side effect is burnout. Their attitude may change from caring and positive to negative and detached.

Studies have shown that caregivers of people with ASD experience higher levels of burnout than caregivers of people with other disabilities. It is likely due to the unique nature of autism, which causes communication and social interaction difficulties, as well as repetitive behaviors, that makes it so much more stressful. A caregiver for a parapalegic will still be able to ask their charge what they want or need at any given time and get a clear answer. This often isn't the case with ASD, and it will take a lot more patience to diagnose a problem and find the right solution.

Caregivers usually feel guilty if they spend time on themselves rather than their children. Many fail to recognize when they are suffering burnout and eventually become incapable of functioning correctly. The burnout related to caring for someone with autism can also take a toll on your health. You may feel isolated, overwhelmed, and anxious.

Finding ways to cope with these feelings and getting support from others is imperative. Many online and in-person support groups for caregivers of people with autism are available. These groups provide valuable information and emotional support. Additionally, many programs and services are available to help people with autism and their caregivers. These resources make the challenges of caregiving more manageable.

What Are the Effects of Caregiver Burnout?

Caregivers should be aware of the toll their role can take on their personal well-being. They often neglect their own physical, spiritual, and emotional well-being because they're too busy caring for others. They're more likely to experience symptoms of depression or anxiety and be at risk of diabetes and heart disease from lack of exercise and a balanced diet. This can lead to developing acute stress-related health issues and depression-like symptoms, such as:

- Withdrawal from family, friends, and social activities
- Suffering depression and anxiety
- Martial issues
- Changes in appetite and weight fluctuations
- Insomnia or changes in sleeping habits
- Increased instances of ill health

- Feeling overwhelmed emotionally, mentally, or physically
- Increased anger or irritability
- Alcohol or drug abuse

These symptoms are compounded by the strain of trying to prevent the person being cared for from experiencing their own negative consequences of ASD. It can quickly spiral out of control if the symptoms are not addressed. Especially in cases where a caregiver is dealing with someone with a severe case of ASD, burnout rates are staggeringly high. When you are working as a professional caregiver, this will invariably have a negative effect on your career and financial stability, while parents and family members often don't have the ability to simply quit their role as a caregiver. Identifying and addressing issues of caregiver burnout will improve things for you and your charges.

CHAPTER FOUR

SELF-CARE STRATEGIES FOR PARENTS OF CHILDREN WITH ASD

Receiving the news that your child was diagnosed with autism spectrum disorders can be a very emotional moment. You will inevitably be thinking about the implications on your child's life, your life, and your relationship with your surroundings. Indeed, it is a turning point in your life. Adjusting to this new reality can take time, and it's a learning process. You won't get everything right from the first moment, and that's okay.

Parenting an autistic child has numerous challenges, starting with the moment your child is diagnosed with ASD. It's something that will affect them for the rest of their life, and inform every decision you make as a parent when raising them. Caring for a child with ASD comes with all the typical challenges of raising a child, and your primary goal as a parent remains the same: keep them safe and healthy, and give them the tools needed to live a happy and successful life. However, ASD adds an extra layer of difficulty to the matter that parents of neurotypical children won't ever have to worry about.

Parenting a child with ASD can be exhausting, and extreme demands will be placed upon your time. In your role as both a parent and caregiver, a great deal will be expected of you emotionally, physically, and psychologically. Because of this, it's easy to focus so much on caring for your child that you ignore your own needs entirely. This can end up being detrimental to your child in the long run. Your health could decline to the point that you can no longer care for your child, and that will end up harming both them *and* you.

The task set before you can feel overwhelming, and that's perfectly natural. It's important to remember that you aren't alone, and there are many parents out there who have been successful in raising a child with ASD. Everyone develops their own way of coping with their new reality, and you will, too. Ultimately, you'll feel a sense of acceptance and do everything in your power to care for your child, sparing no expense or effort to be the best parent possible. When facing the day-to-day challenges as a parent, it's incredibly useful to maintain a healthy self-care regimen for yourself.

How to Care for Yourself as a Parent

The goal here is to keep you mentally, emotionally, and

physically healthy. Anxiety can often be self-perpetuating, and once it gets a foothold, it can be very difficult to break free from the cycle. Parenting a child with ASD is just as much about making sure you can provide them with the best care possible by keeping your body and mind healthy. Here are some ways you can deal with stress and practice healthy self-care:

Understand Fatigue

As a parent of a special needs child, it's vital to take time to reflect on your level of exhaustion. It's easy to get stuck believing you can do it all, but if you neglect your mental, emotional, and physical health, the ramifications can be drastic without realizing it until it's too late.

Take a minute to assess your fatigue levels by asking yourself the following questions:

- Do you feel excessively tired throughout the day?
- Did you have a restless night's sleep?
- Did you sleep enough to deal with daily life responsibilities?
- Create a plan to care for yourself if the answers to these questions indicate fatigue.

Determine What Causes You Stress as a Parent

Children are a handful, even at the best of times. Are they picky eaters? Do they tend to make a mess? Are they throwing temper tantrums that go on for what feels like ages? Make a list of every situation that has caused you anxiety. Break each item on the list down, laying out a flow chart of cause and effect. When the root cause of the stress is laid out right in front of you, it's easier to find a solution that you may not think of when you're in the middle of the situation. Analyzing a problem with a calm, logical mind after you've gotten some distance will avoid the trap of making snap decisions influenced by mounting stress.

Spend Time with Fellow Parents of Children with ASD

Caring for a child with ASD can cause you to lose interest in everything that makes you joyful. But negativity will only make your health worse. It isn't always easy to talk to friends or family members about your struggles if they haven't actually lived the experience of raising a child with ASD. Find parents in a similar situation to your own and make a point to go out to eat or see a movie together. Whether you find talking about these problems to be useful, or simply want a few hours to occupy your mind with something else, there's a good chance another parent out there is feeling the exact same way.

Take a Quick Break

Every parent feels, at one point or another, like breaking everything in sight and screaming at the top of their lungs. Again, you should know that you're not alone. The stress associated with parenthood is very real. Every good parent will most certainly suffer from this one way or another. However, you should resist the urge to let out your anger and remain as calm and composed as possible. Anger, not unlike happiness, is a feeling that comes and goes. Whenever you feel angry, take a step back and a moment to relax. It will soon go away, and you'll go about your life. Remember, the angrier you are, the harder it is to correctly decide regarding your life as well as your child's.

When you are losing your cool, ask a family member or partner to look after your child for a few moments while you step out. You can go to a separate room, watch, or read something funny, or go for a short walk outside the house. When necessary, seek assistance. There will always be things out of your control; don't dwell too much on those. Instead, focus on the things you can change. When you have a clear vision of what you can do, you will be much more composed and will not become consumed with anger and frustration.

While taking a break, try redirecting your attention to something else. Count in reverse from 100 to one. The goal is to divert your attention away from the current circumstance and redirect it to counting those numbers backward. If you're still nervous after the countdown, increase it from 200 to one. Count until you reach a state of tranquility.

Encourage Socialization

It can be hard for a child with ASD to make friends, as they may not pick up on social cues or body language as easily as neurotypical children. However, you should encourage them to try to make friends, be it other children with ASD or otherwise. This doesn't just benefit them, though—if your child spends time with their friends, it can offer you a reprieve for a little while. If your child becomes friends with other children with ASD, you can take turns with the other parents on hosting playdates, trading off giving your fellow parents a break every now and then.

Seeing Family

Invariably, you will do your best to build trust and ensure a safe comfort zone for your child at home. Try to extend this to your family. Most of us feel safe around our families, at least with certain family members. Your child could develop the same comfortable and strong relationships with their extended family.

At some point, many children with ASD will recognize that there is something different about them, and that they feel different from most people. It can be further amplified when they're often isolated and don't spend much time with people other than their parents and siblings. They will feel more appreciated when they see their grandparents, aunts, uncles, and cousins and get their attention. In addition, they will have a lot of fun with their younger relatives and receive gifts from their older ones.

Allowing your child to feel safe and comfortable around their extended family helps immensely with their self-esteem and removes some of your pressure. When your child feels comfortable enough to spend an extended period of time with other members of your family, it can give you a chance to have some time for yourself while they forge a bond with one another.

Don't Be Too Hard on Yourself

It is common for a parent of a child with ASD to feel bad about themselves. It can be as easy as observing that your child does not seem to be improving. As a result, you'll feel guilty and think you are not doing enough to care for them.

If this is your train of thought, you probably are doing more than enough. As long as you give your child all the time in the world and do your best to tend to their needs, there is no reason you should feel this way. Instead of blaming yourself for everything, feel proud of what you are doing. It's never easy to care for an ASD child, and you should appreciate the effort you make every day.

Think of it this way: if you have a close friend with an autistic child, you'll stand by and support them in any way you can. Well, do the same for you.

Keep a Positive Attitude

Like in the classic *Monty Python and the Holy Grail*, you

should always look on the bright side of life, even in the most difficult times. At any given point, you should take the time to reflect on how far you have come and already achieved. Let this give you all the motivation you need to keep going and take care of your child in the best possible way.

Never expect everything to be solved immediately. When faced with difficulties, see them as challenges that must be overcome, and always remember that things can, and will, take time. By managing your expectations and realizing that everything cannot be perfect, you will appreciate the little victories—you will have plenty of those—and stay positive regarding the challenges yet to come.

Educate Your Support System

We can't stress enough how important it is to educate your support system about children with ASD. This applies to your partner, children, family, and friends. By informing people of what it is like to have a child with ASD, you ensure they will be more understanding and compassionate. Your child will encounter many people who have little to no experience with ASD. Inform them of the behavioral issues they might witness and what you do to alleviate these issues. You will be surprised by how much people can be of help in this regard.

Whatever you do, don't keep everything to yourself. Be

open to people; soon enough, you'll be surprised by how much they will be willing to help. Creating and maintaining a supportive environment will take a lot of burdens off your shoulders. The people that care about you, whether family or friends, will adjust and provide significant support.

By creating and maintaining a strong and supportive network, you can rest assured that your child's behavior will never come as a surprise to anyone. Even the younger ones are very perceptive and will know how to interact with your child. Slowly, you will trust more and more people to deal with your child appropriately.

When the people you trust are aware of your everyday struggles, you can be open with them and share your feelings, knowing they will perfectly understand what you are going through. Just like you would support a friend in times of need, you can ensure they will be there for you whenever possible.

Get a Hobby

Do you like playing video games? Maybe you enjoy knitting? Having a hobby you can use to help you take a break from your responsibilities for a little while and do something enjoyable just for yourself isn't selfish, even if your child requires a high degree of hands-on attention. Sometimes, you may not be able to indulge in your hobbies until after they've gone to bed, but make sure to reserve some time to do the things that bring you joy and ease your stress.

Spend Time with Your Partner

Take a trip to the movies together or go for a walk together holding hands. Do housework as a team; it will assist you in bonding and feeling cherished. Knowing that the war is not only your responsibility lifts your spirits and makes your load feel lighter. As humans, we are emotional beings, and we can demonstrate superpowers when our emotions are in good shape. So, spending quality time with your spouse will help boost your mood.

Get Respite Care

If you are the primary caregiver for an autistic child, you will inevitably experience a mental breakdown at some point. Your child will need to be looked after by someone else, like a temporary replacement caregiver, while you recover. This will negatively affect your child, so make sure to ask for assistance if you find yourself in need of it.

Taking care of yourself while also caring for a child with autism is a challenging and time-consuming task. You have a full-time job and a life to live, the child needs money for treatment sessions, and you need money to take care of the child. On top of that, you have many other responsibilities. Ultimately, finding a middle ground and striking a balance is essential. Take it one step at a time, and only accomplish as much as you can each day. If you are the primary caregiver for your child, you must first prioritize maintaining your own physical, emotional, and mental health to provide the best possible care for your child. A kid with autism spectrum disorder cannot be cured, but if the condition is properly managed, the child will mature into an adult capable of doing a great deal for themselves.

Caregiving Responsibilities and Self-Care

Part of practicing good self-care is making your parenting responsibilities as easy on you as possible. As you learn more about how your child responds to certain stimuli and the general habits that they form, you can streamline your caregiving by taking advantage of the experiences relayed by those who have been in your shoes and succeeded.

Create a Routine

Autistic children thrive on repetition. They enjoy doing the same thing over and over, so take advantage of creating a fixed schedule for all your child's activities, such as mealtime, school, therapy, and bedtime. Stick to this framework, and if anything causes you to miss any, inform your child ahead of time so their mind is prepared.

Accept the Autistic Child for Who They Are

Comparing the special needs child to their siblings or other children and expecting them to measure up will not benefit the child. Recognize and accept your child for who they are. Every autistic child, like every neurotypical child, is unique. So, don't expect your child to behave like another person's child merely because they have the same condition. Care for your child's individual needs, and they will bond with you and develop more effectively.

Be Patient and Consistent with Your Child

Children with autism do not learn quickly, and when they do, it is difficult for them to apply what they have learned in a different situation. Your child might learn to welcome at a therapy session or at school, but they don't realize it is vital to greet at home. You must become involved in their activities. Understand what they are being taught to assist your child in replicating the behaviors outside of the environment where it was learned. Interact with your child regularly and assist them in overcoming any obstacles that arise.

Plan Your Child's Meal in Advance

Children can be finicky eaters, but an autistic child is usually even more so. Take your time experimenting to discover what foods your child likes and prepare accordingly - spice up the food to provide a healthy, well-balanced diet. As the child progresses through the developmental stages, observe, and provide what they enjoy eating at each period. Do not force them to eat, as that can lead to an unhealthy relationship with food later in life, sometimes manifesting as eating disorders.

Reward Your Child

Reward your child when they perform well at something. It will encourage more of these behaviors. Target these moments, and instantly praise the child. Children with ASD need to know what they did well so they can replicate this behavior, so make it obvious what earned them the reward. It does not have to be extravagant; a comic book or toy can suffice. When they learn a new skill or complete schoolwork, praise them and always explain why they are being praised.

After completing an activity or basic task, such as finishing their food, brushing their teeth, or cleaning their room, be sure to reward your child as well. It can be simple verbal praise, a hug, or giving them a small treat, like a sticker or piece of candy. This helps to reinforce positive behavior, normalizing it as part of the routine, and makes them more likely to do these activities or tasks without prompting in the future.

Figure Out the Best Way to Communicate

Communicating with your autistic child is exceptionally difficult initially, but once you figure out what works for both of you, it becomes second nature. Before your child communicates effectively, experiment with different communication methods, such as utilizing your eyes, body movements, tone of voice, and how you touch the child. When you and your child can communicate effectively through nonverbal ways, your bond will become stronger.

Study the nonverbal cues used by neurodivergent children to communicate. Examine the child's facial expressions, sounds, and how they appear when stressed, hungry, or requesting something. When you can't figure out what an autistic youngster is saying or frustrated about, the usual reaction is to throw a tantrum. When this occurs, attempt to identify, and resolve the underlying reason for the tantrum. The child thrives best when the link develops stronger and healthier.

Create a Safe Haven at Home

Create a safe haven for the child at home where they can feel secure, safe, and relaxed. To indicate danger zones, use colored tape. Set limits and make them understandable to the child. If your child frequently throws tantrums, carve in precautionary measures to keep the child safe. This zone should have the right color combination to help calm your child down. Allow the child to become acquainted with the safe zone, which will eventually become their favorite place.

Encourage Them to Play

Playing is essential for a child's growth, and autistic children are no exception. Make time to take them to the playground and play with them. It is also an excellent opportunity to bond with your child, so make the most of it. Discover what makes the child feel free and comfortable, what makes them laugh and smile, and provide this content during playtime. Make the child understand that this is an enjoyable time, and they can be free to express themselves while exploring the entire play area.

Have a Treatment Plan

Numerous treatments are available for autism spectrum conditions, and it may be tough to choose one, but keep in mind that each child is unique. What is effective for one autistic child might not be effective for another. While bonding with your child and learning what works and does not work for them is crucial for their development. You must first understand your child's particular needs by confirming what they enjoy, their lacking abilities, and their ideal way to learn (action, seeing, or listening) to create an effective treatment plan.

After determining what works best for your child, be available during their treatment. Your presence encourages the child to respond positively to the therapy. If your mental, emotional, and physical health is in disarray, you will be unable to help your child. So, take care of yourself first so that you adequately care for your child.

CHAPTER FIVE

SELF-CARE STRATEGIES FOR CAREGIVERS OF ADULT OR ELDERLY INDIVIDUALS WITH ASD

Self-care isn't just overlooked by parents, but also caregivers of adults or elderly individuals with ASD. There are unique challenges when serving as this type of primary caregiver, especially on a day-to-day basis. Without possessing the parental authority intrinsic to a child with ASD, caregivers for adults can have a harder time getting their charges to listen to them or cooperate. As a result, caregivers can feel overwhelmed, stressed, and exhausted. Just like with parents, your physical and emotional well-being is essential to care for adults with ASD effectively.

Caring for Yourself

The issues you will face when caring for an adult or elderly individual with ASD become more complex as they age. Unfortunately, this goes the same for you. The types of long hours and physically-demanding work that often accompanies caregiving is much easier to handle when you're in your early 20s, but by the time you're in your 40s and older, your body requires more to keep it running smoothly. People with ASD tend to be set in their ways, and if you take over as their primary caregiver, you will need to figure out how to adjust their routines to suit your responsibilities without causing unnecessary anguish to them. The self-care you practice can be the difference between success and failure, especially when facing the prospect of burnout.

Talk to a Therapist

Caregivers experience high levels of stress on a daily basis, and it will sometimes become necessary to find professional help to aid you in managing that kind of pressure. Talking to a therapist can be an effective method of alleviating the stress you're feeling, especially ones who specialize in treating patients with high stress jobs.

Therapists can provide you with an objective perspective. People can often lose sight of the obvious once they become mired in the minutia of a situation, and it helps to have someone look at things with fresh eyes. They can also offer you helpful coping and problem-solving strategies. Moreover, therapists serve as a sounding board for caregivers who need to vent their frustrations, but either don't have anyone to do that with in their personal life, or would prefer not to dump their problems on a friend or family member.

Yoga

Practicing yoga helps caregivers find a sense of balance and calm in the midst of their busy lives. Yoga helps improve flexibility and strength, which are important when caring for someone with autism. It also helps improve focus and concentration, which is helpful when managing challenging behaviors. There are many different yoga styles, and certain asanas (yoga poses) are particularly helpful for caregivers. For example, the Supported Child's Pose helps calm the nervous system, while the Cat-Cow Pose releases tension in the back and shoulders. In addition, yoga helps reduce stress and anxiety, which are common among caregivers. Yoga practices can provide caregivers with the tools to effectively care for their loved ones while maintaining their physical and mental health.

Reading

First, reading provides a much-needed break from the demands of caregiving. It is usually difficult to find time for yourself when you're caring for someone with autism, but reading can give you a chance to relax and recharge. In addition, reading can also help you learn more about autism and how best to care for someone with the condition. A wealth of books is available on the subject, so you can find one that meets your needs and interests. When you're feeling stressed or overwhelmed, it's easy to unwind and decompress when you disappear into the pages of a book.

Second, reading helps to take your mind off your problems and responsibilities when you aren't "on the clock." It can be difficult to simply stop thinking about the many things you must do the next day, but never getting a break from that can take a toll on your mental and physical health. Reading can provide a welcome respite from the challenges of caregiving and reduce stress levels. Studies have shown that reading lowers blood pressure and heart rate and reduces the stress hormone cortisol level.

Join Dance Classes

Dance is a great way to get your body moving, have some fun, and be an excellent form of exercise. With different dance classes available, you can certainly find one that suits your interests and fitness level.

Dance classes are also a great way to meet new people and socialize. These classes are wonderful ways to connect with like-minded people if you feel isolated. Still, if you cannot join a dance class, you can always put on some music and create your own dance moves at home to unwind.

Remain Consistent

It is easy to let go of your daily rituals when you feel overwhelmed, but sticking to them as much as possible is essential. Whether making time for breakfast in the morning or reading a book before bed, these rituals will help bring a sense of normalcy to your day. Eat your meals at regular times; it will create structure and balance for you and your child. These small things can make a big difference to your overall well-being.

Make Time for Yourself

It is important for parents to make time for themselves, even if it is just a few minutes each day. Use this time for activities, such as reading, listening to music, or taking a relaxing bath. Doing something you enjoy reduces stress levels and improves your mood.

Getting up 30 minutes earlier each day or taking a break while your child is napping will enable you to fit some "me time" into your daily routine. If you have difficulty finding time for yourself, ask a friend or family member to watch your child for a few hours to have some time for yourself.

Indulge in Crafting

Crafting can be a relaxing and stress-relieving activity. It is also a fun activity to do with your child. The different crafts you can do are endless, such as painting, knitting, or scrapbooking. Children with autism are often very creative, so you could find that they enjoy crafting tremendously. So, together you can create some cherished memories and bond as a family.

Connect with Nature

Spending time in nature helps boosts your mood and reduces stress levels. Even if you live in an urban area, there are likely to be parks or green spaces nearby you can visit.

Spend time in nature daily; a walk in the park, sitting in your garden, or even just looking out the window at the trees. If you have a pet, playing with them outdoors is also beneficial for you and your pet.

Open up about How You're Feeling

For most parents, it isn't easy to talk about how you're feeling, but communicating with your partner or a close friend about what you're going through is essential. Bottling up your emotions can lead to isolation and despair. You have additional responsibilities and stresses that many people cannot understand. So, for the benefit of your well-being, allocate some time each week to discuss how you're doing, both good and bad.

Seek Professional Help If Needed

If your child's diagnosis causes unbearable stress, seeking professional help is crucial for your mental and physical health. A mental health professional provides support and guidance on coping with your child's ASD.

Take a Break

There will be times when you feel like you can't do it

anymore. So, it is vital to take a break before you reach your breaking point. It can be a day, a weekend, or even longer if needed.

Ask your close friends or family to care for your child so you can take the time for yourself. Use this time to relax and recharge. You can't pour from an empty cup, so make sure to take care of yourself first. Don't assume it is selfish to take time for yourself. You need to care for yourself to be the best parent for your ASD child.

Seek Help from Others

There is no shame in admitting that you need help. Many resources are available in-person or online to parents of children with ASD. Talk to your child's doctor or a mental health professional for advice on getting started.

ASD is a difficult diagnosis for parents to cope with, but with a good support system, you can work wonders. You can seek help from your local autism organizations. These organizations provide you with information and resources on ASD. There are many helpful websites and books available, too.

Have Realistic Expectations

Raising a child with ASD can be stressful and overwhelming at times. Therefore, it is also important to accept that there will be challenges. ASD is a lifelong condition, so it is best to accept that there will be good and bad days. Although challenging, focus on the positive aspects of your child's ASD. For example, many children with ASD are extremely creative and have unique perspectives of the world. There are many similar examples; reaching out to others will expose you to them.

One Day at a Time

One of the best pieces of advice for parents of children with ASD is to take things one day at a time. This can be difficult, but it is important to remember that progress is often slow.

Do not compare your child's progress to other children's, and do not compare your parenting to other parents. Every child and every family is different, so what works for one does not always work for another.

Remember, children with ASD do not "grow out of" their diagnosis. While they learn to cope with their symptoms and lead happy, fulfilling lives, ASD is a lifelong condition.

Acceptance

It is important to accept your child for who they are. ASD is a part of your child and should not be seen as negative or debilitating. Embrace your child's differences and help them grow into the best person they can be. Your support will help them reach their full potential. Your love and care will ensure them that they are a little different but never less in your eyes.

Caring for yourself is essential for parents of children with ASD. By following these tips, you will reduce stress, maintain your energy levels, and be the best parent possible. Like every responsible parent, you want the best for your child, and by considering your health and well-being, you ensure that your child has the best possible life.

CHAPTER SIX

CARING FOR YOUR LONG-TERM HEALTH

Eat a Healthy Diet

Eating a healthy diet is important for everyone, but it is especially significant for parents and caregivers of children with autism. Eating healthy foods ensures more energy to deal with challenging behaviors.

You might find it difficult to eat a healthy diet as an adult with autism. You could have trouble preparing meals or dislike the taste of certain foods. However, it is important to eat various healthy foods to get the nutrients your body needs.

Some Tips for Healthy Eating

Here are some tips for eating a healthy diet as an adult who cares for children with autism:

Plan Ahead

Meal planning will help you eat a healthy diet. Planning your meals in advance makes you less likely to make unhealthy choices. You do not have much time to cook as a busy parent or caregiver. Meal planning will help you save time and money.

You can make meal planning easier by batch cooking, meaning cooking a large amount of food at once and storing it in the freezer. When you are ready to eat, you can just reheat the food. It is a great time saver.

You can batch cook healthy meals, such as stews, soups, and casseroles on the weekend and freeze them. You will have healthy meals ready to eat during the week.

Eat Breakfast

Starting your day with a healthy breakfast can give you the energy you need to care for your child with autism. If you don't have a habit of eating breakfast, start slowly by eating a piece of fruit or yogurt. Once you get into the habit of eating breakfast, you can add more items to your breakfast, such as oatmeal, eggs, or toast.

You can also eat many breakfast foods on the go, such as granola bars, muffins, or yogurt. Or prepare over-the-night oats so you can just grab them and go in the morning.

Make Time to Eat

It is important to make time to eat, even if you are busy. If you do not have time to sit down and eat a meal, snack on healthy foods throughout the day. Eating several small meals throughout the day is better than skipping them.

Skipping meals can make you tired and irritable. When you are tired, it is harder to deal with challenging behaviors.

Pack Healthy Snacks

Packing healthy snacks when you are out and about will help you avoid unhealthy choices. Some healthy snack ideas include:

- Fresh fruit or vegetables
- Yogurt
- Whole grain crackers
- Trail mix
- Granola bars
- Hard-boiled eggs

Drink Plenty of Fluids

Drinking plenty of fluids is vital for everyone, but it is particularly vital for caregivers of children with autism. When you are well-hydrated, you will have more energy and think more clearly.

You will find it difficult if you are not used to drinking enough fluids. However, there are many ways to ensure you get enough fluids.

Some Tips for Drinking Enough Fluids

Drink Water Throughout the Day: Carry a water bottle with you and drink water throughout the day.

Drink Other Fluids: In addition to water, you can also

drink other fluids, such as juice, milk, and herbal tea.

Eat Foods with High Water Content: Eating certain foods with a high water content helps you stay hydrated. Some examples of foods with a high water content include:

- Watermelon
- Strawberries
- Oranges
- Cucumbers

Avoid Sugary Drinks: Sugary drinks like soda and energy drinks make you feel tired and irritable. It is best to avoid these drinks and stick to water and other healthy choices.

Avoid Processed Foods

Processed foods are high in sugar, salt, and fat. They also contain chemicals that are not good for your health. Eating processed foods leads to weight gain, high blood pressure, and type 2 diabetes.

As a caregiver of a child with autism, you may be tempted to eat processed foods because they are easy to prepare. However, it is important to eat healthy foods as much as possible.

Tips for Avoiding Processed Foods

- **Read Food Labels:** When grocery shopping, read the food labels to see how processed the food is. The more ingredients a food has, the more processed it is. Also, check the sugar and fat content of the food. Choose foods with few ingredients and are low in sugar and fat.

- **Eat Whole Foods**: Whole foods are unprocessed and often healthier than processed foods. Examples of whole foods include fruits, vegetables, and whole grains.

- **Prepare Meals from Scratch:** Cooking meals from scratch help you avoid processed foods. Preparing meals from scratch takes more time, but it is worth the effort. Also, you will know what is in your food precisely and control the amount of sugar, salt, and fat.

- **Get Your Child Involved in Meal Planning and Preparation:** Getting your autistic child involved in meal planning and preparation is a great way to teach them about healthy eating. It will also make mealtime more enjoyable for everyone.

- **Limit Screen Time:** Too much screen time can lead to unhealthy eating habits. It is vital to limit screen time for children and adults. Set limits on how much time you and your family spend in front of screens.

Tips for Limiting Screen Time

1. Find Other Activities to Do: You and your family can do many other activities instead of watching TV or using electronic devices. Some ideas include playing games, reading books, and going for walks.

2. Make Screen Time Active: If you are watching TV or using electronic devices, make it an active experience. For example, stand up and dance while you watch TV. Or play an active video game, such as Wii bowling.

3. Be a Good Role Model: Children learn by example. You must be a good role model if you want to limit your child's screen time. Turn off the mobile and put away your electronic devices when it is time to do other things.

Create Balance

When there is a disorder in your life, it becomes one of the biggest stresses. Many things are happening at the same time that is not prioritized. You are highly busy but underutilized, and it will devastate you mentally and emotionally. Make a list of everything you need to do every day and rank them in order of importance. Allot time to each point and stick to it to keep order. This routine will ensure that all major aspects of your life receive the necessary attention. Maintaining a sense of balance in your schedule not only lowers your stress but also makes you more productive and happier.

Parents of young kids with autism spectrum disorders (ASDs) reportedly have a higher level of psychological and emotional turmoil than parents with other neurodevelopmental disorders. Most are due to autism-related behavioral patterns like self-mutilation, abuse, and breakdowns, meaning they require a strictly rigid schedule. For parents, these routines are exhausting, frustrating, and even risky. Autism spectrum character traits make it difficult to find competent alternate care, putting more duty on the parents of autistic children than on other disabilities.

Seeking help might even increase a parent's stress levels due to concerns about their children's overall well-being. Trusting substitute care workers is hard for any parent, and autistic parents have far more cause to worry.

Self-Care Is Not Selfishness

Originally, the term "self-care" was used to refer to someone dealing with a long-term illness. Participating in their medication and treatment regimen rather than relying solely on medical professionals has significantly improved health outcomes and allowed people to live longer regardless of their circumstances. Self-care has changed much over the years. It is presently seen as a way of minimizing long-term illness and increasing the average lifespan for every individual.

Self-care encompasses almost anything, from simple necessities like hygiene practices and a nutritious diet to stress-relieving activities, such as mindfulness meditation and even yoga. According to studies, relatives or household caregiving is a serious public health problem attributed to the rising effort and cash required to meet the specific needs of several reliant kids.

A study discovered that parents who cared for severely ill children were more likely to experience chromosomal changes. This accounts for early aging due to abnormally high production of hormones, including stress hormones, norepinephrine, and epinephrine. Putting a stop to that stress, for just a short time, will hugely impact physical and psychological health. Caregivers and parents who manage to minimize their stress levels by taking self-care seriously are capable of living longer than the average life expectancy.

Self-Care Is Easier Said Than Done

As a parent taking care of an autistic child, caring for yourself becomes more challenging than caring for the child. Taking a vacation or choosing a new hobby are simple stress-relieving measures that could also boost the general well-being of an average parent of an autistic child. For instance, sport is said to add roughly a decade to a human's life. Sadly, full-time parent caregivers seldom have the opportunity of engaging in these self-focused practices.

Each family case is unique and different, but the protection of every kid will still take precedence. Even taking a bath can be difficult at times, especially if the autistic child is prone to self-harm or elopement. However, creating even a small amount of breathing space for yourself could do wonders in the quest to improve the entire family's well-being.

Are you the mother or father of an autistic child? Are you struggling physically or mentally? You can take care of yourself by rating yourself based on the following self-care attributes.

Physical Self-Care

How Seriously Do You Take Your Physical Well-Being?

Physical self-care is perhaps the most fundamental and essential self-care you can learn. It could be as basic as cleaning your teeth and taking a nice shower every morning. Once you've mastered physical self-care, it will be much easier for you to form other self-care habits.

Do You Get Adequate Rest?

Do you know that sleep is an important aspect of self-care? You are an adult and should aim to sleep for seven to nine hours every night. It's also critical to get adequate rest in the daytime. This might entail taking multiple rest periods throughout the day so that you can care for your child with more energy and clarity of mind. Do not stay up at night worrying about when you should be sleeping. Not getting sufficient rest might lead to frustration in the long run.

Are You Hydrated and Eating Well?

Do you know that proper nutrition is mostly about finding the right balance? Meals that leave you feeling healthier and cared for are crucial, and so is treating yourself on special occasions. Besides eating well-balanced meals drinking plenty of water during the day is important. Taking good care of the simple necessities might appear straightforward, but they are crucial. It is important not to fall into the habit of eating fast foods and snacks when taking care of your child. Take your time to make proper meal plans for the day or the whole week.

Do You Take Your Emotional Self-Care Seriously?

Emotional self-care includes spending some time recognizing and addressing your emotions, feelings, and behavior patterns. It is also discovering wholesome ways of expressing these feelings, including any behavior used to deal with stress, convey feelings, and cultivate positive emotions regarding life. Do you assume that you know your emotions at any given time? Do you know those unaddressed feelings significantly impact how you think, your decisions, and your interactions with others?

People usually push negative thoughts away to be addressed later or overlook them entirely since they don't want to focus on them. People who do this might discover that they are not as accomplished as they thought and might struggle to learn the underlying reasons. The following are ways to care for yourself while not jeopardizing your child.

Do You Meditate?

Meditation is simply observing the present situation without conviction. Settle in with these feelings and merely breathe. Your thoughts, emotions, and feelings are neither good nor bad, innocent, or guilty; they simply exist. Do you know that letting your feelings emerge is a component of empathy and self-care?

Are You Capable of Choosing Your Reactions with Care?

Even if we can't control what occurs to us, we can control how we react to those events. You always have the option to take deep breaths, react with compassion towards yourself and everyone else, and seek ways to sustain hope and contentment as you deal with your autistic child.

Limit Your Exposure to News

The Centers for Disease Control and Prevention recommends reducing exposure to mainstream media, particularly during challenging times. Take frequent pauses from current events and rather engage in healthy, enjoyable activities.

Are You Maintaining Contact with Others?

Supportive and loving relationships will help you remain secure and emotionally stable. It is far more crucial than ever to stay in contact and keep in touch with others during difficult times. Also, these people can help you take care of your child when you are occupied with other important things or when you need a break.

Are You Capable of Exercising Gratitude?

Switching your attention from what's wrong to what is right is an excellent way of practicing emotional self-care. Do you know that incorporating gratitude into your daily routine greatly improves your overall mental health?

How Often Do You Laugh?

Connect with friends who cheer you up, or binge-watch an entertaining show. Do these things with your children and enjoy quality family time? Do you know that laughter is known to reduce stress and enhance mood? It is even beneficial for innate immunity. Emotional self-care is essential, but it does not have to be intense.

Do You Have a Relaxing Hobby or Pastime?

Do you stitch, crochet, or play the guitar? Perhaps you enjoy painting? Or how about those leisure activities you usually enjoy but have since abandoned? While concentrating on stress relief, enjoyable activities are excellent ways to wind down and relax your mind.

Consider doing these pastime activities with your kid; perhaps they will discover that they love one or two, too.

Consider the following questions when evaluating your emotional self-care approaches:

- Do you still have healthy coping mechanisms for your emotions?
- Do you include practices in your daily life that allow you to replenish?

Do You Practice Spiritual Self-Care?

Spiritual self-care may be religious or non-religious. According to research, a religious or spiritual way of life is usually a happier way of life. Fostering your spirit does not have to entail religion. It can include anything that aids in developing a greater meaning and purpose, comprehension, or link with existence.

Spiritual self-care is essential, whether you relish mindfulness, attend religious services, or say a prayer. Even if it is not usually done properly, most people recognize the significance of caring for their physical and emotional health, but their spiritual self is always overlooked. Whereas spiritual self-care is as crucial as all other areas of self-care. These are how you can care for yourself while also ensuring your child is safe and protected.

How Often Do You Contemplate?

Contemplation entails thinking over something constantly, learning and ruminating about it, normally something noteworthy and crucial relating to life and its significance. When you become very still and extremely focused while pondering, your self-importance partially dissolves, and your contemplation becomes progressively like mindfulness. At these times, answers to your life's challenges can appear unexpectedly.

Have You Been Spending Time in Nature?

Do you know that this is among the ideal spiritual self-care practices you can do to ensure optimum well-being? According to a study, spending quality time in nature reduces stress.

After awakening or experiencing a significant spiritual shift, most people feel compelled to spend more time in nature. Some parts of us long for an ego-free attachment when we open up and work through our problems. It is also one of the activities you can do with your autistic child. Rather than leaving them at home, why not spend time together in nature? You can also grow a garden in your compound, so you won't have to go away from home whenever you need vegetables.

Do You Judge Yourself?

You must know that you are trying your best, you are

doing great, and you should take it easy on yourself. If you've ever been in continuous judgment of yourself, you'll understand that it's a harmful way of living and won't help you develop good emotional and psychological well-being.

Do you know that judgment takes away your ability to sense and obey your spiritual guide? It is a way of measuring up to what is widely accepted, increasing the likelihood to fit in and also be understood, or, in other words, loved. Anxiety about not being appreciated and recognized can cause us to discard and dismiss others to avoid being dismissed and rejected.

Are you submitting to the general and public's thoughts by choosing to live in this manner? Instead of living with forethought of everything you want your life to be, become less judgmental because when you stop judging yourself, you create liberating spiritual values, open to giving and receiving love on many levels. You have a sense of calm and contentment because you are not labeling things or making up a false sense of happiness. Everything should be appreciated for its simple beauty.

While working on your spirituality, answer these questions as they will help you know where you stand.

Do you make time to indulge in something you appreciate, such as painting or crafting, growing vegetables, a pastime, or even a daily diary?

Do you go to a sanctuary, regularly meditate, or find a different way to express your religious views freely? It may be something as simple as reading poetry or praying before dinner.

- Are you able to incorporate laughter into your daily life?

- Do you manage to spend quality time outside?

Growth and Renewal

Are you interested in learning and exploring different things, like new approaches to an issue or new principles that guide things?

Do you also have plans in place to broaden your horizons? It could include new skills and concepts or hobbies, like crocheting or woodwork, reading novels, or watching movies about things that interest you beyond your daily life.

Do you still have aspirations or long-term objectives you have designed small measures to accomplish?

Give detailed answers and consideration to these growth and renewal questions.

Benefits of Long-Term Self-Care for Parents

As an autism caregiver, self-care may seem like a luxury. You're so busy supporting your autistic child and taking care of your other commitments that you don't have much time for anything else. But lately, you've felt exhausted and frustrated. You should be caring for yourself because only when you have good health can you care for your child.

Self-care is essential for your well-being and fulfillment, particularly when combined with the noteworthy challenges associated with raising autistic children. Normal self-practices lay the groundwork for better mental health. It combats detrimental emotions like stress, frustration, and loneliness while also elevating your mood. The following are benefits of self-care for autistic parents.

Self-Care Is Critical for Your Overall Well-Being

You're not only dealing with familiar parenting issues but also assisting your child in coping with the challenges that come with their Asperger's syndrome. These could include dealing with complex sensory sensitivities, temper tantrums, social troubles, and nervousness. Likewise, you are most likely assisting your kid in developing an individualized education program and helping them, so they accomplish their academic and behavioral objectives. Meetings with instructors, advisors, and therapists are usually required.

When the requirements of autism parenthood coincide with their daily hassles, they can become exhausted. They don't have much to give to anyone, including themselves.

They don't even have the time for their very important self-care.

The problem is that you cannot pour from an empty cup. When you fail to care for yourself, you struggle in all aspects of life. You will have difficulty parenting your child while also navigating your daily life. Self-care makes you empathetic to your child while reducing anger and anxiety. Similarly, self-care allows you to be more available and clear-headed, which is essential in dealing with many of the difficulties you face. Therefore, if you take good care of yourself, you will also be best prepared to care for those you love.

Self-Care Is Setting a Great Example for Your Child

If these aren't enough to persuade you, consider the example you're setting for the child. It isn't unusual for neurodivergent people to go to extraordinary lengths to blend in with their colleagues. But they have to conceal their true identity. However, this eventually causes a lot of stress and burnout. Self-care is also essential to their accomplishments. Autistic people require time to recuperate their batteries and regroup. However, they frequently disregard it in the best interests of trying to fit in or being appreciated.

It is critical to demonstrate to your child that you appreciate self-care and recognize its importance to your mental well-being. If a child sees you taking care of yourself, they will also become more inclined to do so.

Ways to Practice Long-Term Self-Care

A seemingly endless supply of self-care tips can be found online. The usual mindfulness techniques seem impossible for parents of special needs children; the idea of dedicating extended periods alone seems like a dream world. Whereas in reality, you have little time to spend alone or possibly none at all if you have a child that needs round-the-clock care. However, it doesn't mean you can't do things to give yourself some much-needed self-love. These won't involve enjoying a sunrise or a perfect Warrior Pose on the beach during sunset.

Meditate

Meditation can help you relieve stress and improve your well-being. The great thing is that it can be practiced anywhere at any time. All you need is to find a comfortable place to sit or lie down and focus on your breath. As you inhale and exhale, keep your mind from wandering by focusing on the sensation of your breath moving in and out of your body. If your mind wanders, simply bring your attention back to your breath. Over time, focusing on your breath and letting go of intrusive thoughts becomes easier. In addition to reducing stress, meditation is known for improving sleep quality, increasing calm and peace, and boosting immunity.

Guided meditation, guided imagery, visualization, and other forms of meditation help manage stress. When you meditate, you focus your attention and clear your mind of racing thoughts. Meditation helps calm and center you, giving you a much-needed break from the constant noise in your head. Guided meditation involves following someone else's voice as they lead you through the process. Guided imagery is similar, but instead of focusing on your breath, you focus on visualizing peaceful images in your mind. Visualization is another effective form of meditation; it involves picturing yourself in a calm, relaxing place and focusing on positive feelings.

So how can you get started? There are many resources available online and in libraries. You can also find mobile apps that offer guidance and support. Once you find a practice that works for you, stick with it. The more you meditate, the more beneficial it can be, especially for caregivers who are often under a lot of strain. With regular meditation practice, caregivers can better manage the challenges of caring for someone with autism while also caring for themselves.

Meditation can help settle a busy mind and tired body. You can incorporate this stress-busting practice into your daily routine in various ways. It helps you re-center your mind and return to the present moment when you feel off-balance or emotionally fraught. It might sound strange if you've never tried it before, but after regular practice, you'll find yourself relying on meditation to enhance your emotional well-being.

As a parent of a special needs child, it's not feasible to retreat into tranquil woods or a picturesque beach in Bali. In this case, try the counting meditation technique. Choose a number - it could be 10 or 100 and just relax, focus, and count. Your mind refocuses on counting, not the stressor. It's the most straightforward method to help with awareness and keeps you grounded in the present.

Don't Keep Things to Yourself

People genuinely care and want to help others who are struggling. Express your feelings to your loved ones. It is emotionally and physically exhausting as the primary caregiver for a child with special needs. Most people probably have no idea how you feel, so don't be afraid to ask for help. All it takes is a listening ear or a few hours away for you to recharge.

Find a local network support group and plan afternoon walks. If you can't leave the house, getting together on a live video chat is a great way to connect with others in the same situation. You might even find that you can help other parents who are lonely.

Alleviate Pressure with Entertainment

All forms of entertainment can increase our dopamine levels. Music is one of the most common methods of achieving this. We are all capable of responding to music. Without doing much more than listening, it can profoundly affect our bodies and brains positively. When things become too overwhelming or you feel your irritability levels spiking, music can help distract you from disturbing thoughts and soothe emotions. Create a playlist with the most positive affirming songs you know, and play them on repeat until you know the lyrics and sing your heart out to relieve stress. Then create a new playlist with slow-tempo songs to help calm nervous emotions.

Films and TV shows can have a similar effect on your brain, but they tend to require more of an investment. However, studies have shown that people who follow a TV series or watch movies regularly have reduced stress, more energy, and high levels of creativity. The enjoyment you get from consuming this type of media is comparable to a night out with friends, as audiences often form parasocial relationships with their favorite characters. While it's not a substitute for real life interactions, gathering friends together for a watch party can be a great way to hang out with others and relax.

Create a To-Do List of Things You Enjoy

Taking care of your children is a rewarding and life-fulfilling experience. However, it can derail your desire to do things you enjoy. Creating a healthy living environment is achieved when everyone is happy, so you need to be doing the activities that bring you joy.

Perhaps it's been too long since you've self-indulged, and to remember those hobbies or activities that made you smile, it's a great idea to create a list of those things and start with the easiest first. It doesn't make you a bad person for wanting things for yourself or desire a non-parent activity for an hour or two or a whole day.

Keep a Health Diary

Health diaries can allow you to keep track of your exercise routines, eating habits, and changes in your overall health. Our bodies rarely change overnight, and because the changes are often incremental, if you aren't keeping a record of it, you may not understand how your health reached a certain point.

Something to remember when keeping a health diary:

Keep it private. Your health and medical history is your own, and you don't have to share them with anyone else. Alternatively, it could help you to communicate your issues without expressing them verbally. How much of your health diary you feel comfortable sharing with others is up to you.

Maintain a routine. A good habit to get into is logging

your meals, including what you eat and how much you eat, immediately after the meal has ended. This will ensure you have the most accurate data possible. Do the same thing with any workouts, noting what specific exercises you did and how many reps of each one. When you notice any changes in your health, be sure to record those in the diary as well.

Make it accessible. Since you'll be using your health diary to track things like meals and exercises, it should be somewhere that you can easily reach in order to record your progress. If you want to use a pen and paper diary, keep it near your kitchen or wherever you normally eat your meals. There are also health diary apps you can download and log all the pertinent information onto your phone. Avoid using post-it notes or loose pieces of paper, as they can get ruined or lost, defeating the purpose of the diary. Buying a traditional logbook may cost a bit more, but since you can use it to keep track of everything in one place, you'll be more likely to use it.

Set yourself health goals. When you start using your health diary, jot down some goals you would like to achieve within the next month, three months, six months, and/or year. Keep them realistic, but choose a target that will require you to push yourself to reach. Whether it's losing weight, lifting a certain amount, being able to run a mile under a specific time, etc., having a goal you need to work toward can be a great motivator to stay on top of your health and continue keeping track of everything.

Some Extra Tips to Stay Healthy in the Long-Term

You do not have to go to extremes to promote long-term self-care. Sometimes, the small things count toward taking care of yourself, but it can be difficult if you are busy caring for others. Ensure you're sticking to the essential aspects of maintaining your well-being:

- Maintain a reasonably active lifestyle by doing specific daily active tasks - morning walk, cardio in the living room, dancing to music.

- Take care of your body by brushing your teeth, taking a shower, and washing your hair.

- Consume well-balanced meals at the same time every day.

- Don't forget to hydrate - coffee doesn't count. At least six glasses of water per day are required for healthy digestion and other critical bodily functions.

- Keep up with cleanliness. It can be challenging to maintain your house with so much going on, but putting things away as soon as you're finished with them will help long-term.

CHAPTER SEVEN

COPING WITH ASD-RELATED STRESS

Stress and anxiety are major factors in caregivers suffering physically, mentally, and emotionally. It can also be difficult to cope with the demands placed upon you, especially if you are the sole caregiver. Unsurprisingly, many caregivers of individuals with ASD experience increased levels of depression, anxiety, and other psychological distress. The longer stress and anxiety goes untreated, the more volatile the reaction will be when it finally overwhelms you.

Think of it like a bottle of soda—if you continuously shake it, pressure will keep building up inside, and if it isn't released, it will eventually cause the bottle to explode. You need to find methods to allow that pressure to vent periodically to avoid an explosion. This doesn't even necessarily mean erupting into a fit of anger. Untreated stress and anxiety can manifest in a number of different ways, but all are detrimental to your health.

Types of Stress Experienced by Parents and Caregivers

Psychological Distress

Several factors can contribute to psychological stress. First, caring for a person with autism often requires a great deal of time and energy. Parents and caregivers easily become overwhelmed between therapy appointments, school meetings, and everyday caregiving tasks. In addition, the financial costs can be significant. Many families find themselves struggling to pay for treatment and support services, adding even more stress to an already challenging situation.

Furthermore, dealing with the public perception of autism is not easy and also very frustrating. Although increased awareness has led to a greater understanding of the condition, there is still stigma attached to autism, making it harder for parents and caregivers to feel like they have the support they need. When faced with all these challenges, it's no wonder many parents and caregivers of children with autism experience increased levels of depression, anxiety, or other psychological distress.

Symptoms of Psychological Distress

As a caregiver, being aware of the signs of psychological distress is important. It is a condition that occurs when someone is dealing with a lot of stress and can seriously impact your mental and physical health. Symptoms of psychological distress include feeling overwhelmed, exhausted, or hopeless. You might also find yourself withdrawing from activities you once enjoyed, or you have difficulty concentrating or sleeping. If you experience any of these symptoms, it's important to reach out for help. Many resources are available to caregivers struggling with psychological distress, and getting support will significantly impact your well-being.

Physical Stress

Being a caregiver includes many physical demanding requirements. This can be anything from restraining someone who is lashing out and liable to hurt themselves or others, to staying awake and alert with very little sleep because the person in your care needs attention from you. Unfortunately, this constant stress will take a toll on your health. Studies have shown that caregivers of individuals with ASD are more likely to suffer from cardiovascular, immune system, and gastrointestinal problems. In addition, the physical demands of caregiving make it challenging to get enough sleep, exercise, and eat a healthy diet, further exacerbating the effects of stress.

You also suffer from increased fatigue or struggle with insomnia, especially if you have a young child with ASD who struggles with sleep. While it's important to get enough rest, it is not easy when you're constantly worrying about your child's health and safety. Stress from lack of sleep becomes compounded as you go consecutive days without proper rest, and can severely affect your problem-solving and decision-making abilities.

Symptoms Indicating Physical Stress

One of the most common symptoms of physical stress is an elevated heart rate. When you're under a lot of physical stress by managing constant demands and problems with autistic children, our bodies release a hormone called cortisol. Cortisol helps us deal with short-term threats by increasing our heart rate and blood pressure and giving us a burst of energy. However, if we're constantly stressed, our bodies can't keep up with the demand for cortisol, and it will take a toll on our health.

One of the most common symptoms of physical stress is an elevated heart rate. When you're under a lot of physical stress by managing constant demands and problems with autistic children, your body releases a hormone called cortisol. Cortisol helps us to deal with short-term threats by increasing our heart rate and blood pressure and giving us a burst of energy.

However, if we're constantly stressed, our bodies can't keep up with the demand for cortisol, which takes a toll on our health. One of the most common symptoms of physical stress is persistent thoughts about one or more stressors because cortisol affects the part of the brain responsible for decision-making and long-term planning. When physically stressed, we focus on the things that cause anxiety rather than thinking about ways to solve the problem. As a result, we end up feeling overwhelmed and hopeless.

If you have trouble shaking off stress-related thoughts, it's important to take notice.

If left unchecked, physical stress leads to serious health problems like heart disease and depression. Fatigue is another symptom of physical stress that has many causes. It could be the result of overexertion, lack of sleep, or an underlying medical condition. In addition, stress interferes with sleep, which also contributes to fatigue. If you're feeling fatigued, it may be worth evaluating your stress levels and making some changes to reduce stress.

Societal Stress

Stress in relation to autism doesn't just come from the individuals with ASD. In addition to tackling the challenges of managing ASD daily, you also have to contend with the misconceptions and lack of understanding from society at large. There is a stigma around people with ASD, and while it has improved in recent years, there are still many people who simply don't comprehend the reality of living with it. This can lead to isolation and constant anxiety for caregivers. You may feel you have to justify your decisions to friends and family members who don't have firsthand experience with autism. As a result, it's not surprising that societal stress is a major issue for caregivers, especially parents.

However, there are ways to cope with societal stress. Seek support from other parents and caregivers, educate yourself about autism, and advocate for a better understanding and acceptance from society. With the right support network, you can find ways to cope with societal stress. Seek support from other parents and caregivers, educate yourself about autism, and advocate for better understanding and acceptance from society. With the right support network, you can manage the societal stress that comes with being an autistic parent or caregiver.

Symptoms of Societal Stress

You might be wondering what societal stress is and how it differs from everyday stressors. Societal stress refers to the cumulative effect of various environmental factors on an individual's mental and physical health. These factors can include economic insecurity, social isolation, discrimination, constantly judged, problem interaction, and exposure to violence. While some degree of stress is inevitable, chronic stress can lead to serious health problems such as anxiety, depression, heart disease, and stroke.

Symptoms of Societal Stress manifest in a variety of ways. For some people, it manifests as physical symptoms like headaches or stomach aches. Others may experience difficulty sleeping or concentrating or feel highly anxious or irritable. Some people turn to alcohol or drugs to cope with societal stress, while others withdraw from friends and family. If you regularly experience any of these symptoms, it is important to seek help from a mental health professional. With treatment, you can learn healthy coping mechanisms and manage your stress more positively.

Financial Stress

Although we spoke a little bit about the financial pressure faced by caregivers, it's worth addressing the stress caused by these financial issues in more detail. There are substantial costs for therapy and treatment, adapting your home for an individual with ASD, and accommodating any other special needs required for caregiving. Sometimes this means buying medical equipment or other tools to help ease the burden on the individual with ASD. Between medical bills, therapy costs, and specialized education, the expenses can quickly add up.

Some government programs may offer assistance, but they generally won't cover the full cost of essential care. As a result, many parents are left struggling to make ends meet. In some cases, they are even forced to choose between paying for their child's care and meeting basic needs. Unfortunately, government benefits or insurance do not always alleviate the financial strain. In many cases, parents have to shoulder the burden, leading to immense financial strain and emotional stress.

ASD caregiver support groups often host special events like playdates and birthday parties that provide valuable opportunities for social interaction. Similarly, you have to spend on specialized and costly equipment like weighted blankets, interactive media tablets, and sensory toys, which help your child regulate their environment and behavior. Although they cost more upfront, these investments pay off in the long run by helping your child lead a happy and healthy life. Unfortunately, at the same time, they can dent your budget.

Due to communication issues, it's not always easy to determine when a person with ASD is having a negative reaction to the typical stimuli that triggers outbursts, or if they are suffering from some other kind of ailment that they simply can't explain effectively. This can lead to parents making additional trips to the doctor or hospital in order to have a doctor perform a checkup when it turns out there wasn't actually a health issue. Conversely, if a potential illness or ailment is mistaken for regular ASD-related problems, getting medical care might not happen until the ailment has progressed, necessitating more expensive treatment.

There are a few things that you can do to try to ease the financial burden. Firstly, ensure to apply for all the government benefits and programs you could be eligible for. Secondly, talk to your employers about flexible work arrangements or other accommodations that might help you balance your work and caregiving responsibilities. Thirdly, reach out to friends and family members for help and support. Remember, you are not alone in this – many other parents are in similar situations. There is strength in numbers, so don't hesitate to ask for help when needed.

Tips for Overcoming Stress

Change Your Routine

You don't always have to implement major alterations to your life in order to reduce stress. There are simple changes you can make to your routine that can be very effective in managing the anxiety brought on by the challenges of being a caregiver. If the person you're caring for wakes up at roughly the same time each day, try waking up an hour earlier. This will allow you some time to mentally prepare for the day, eat some breakfast, and have a cup of coffee. Because of the way our brains handle the transition from a state of rest, there can be a period where you feel groggy and muddled. Immediately jumping into your caregiver duties after waking up can be taxing on your mind, starting your day with a stressful experience.

Another helpful strategy is to coordinate windows of opportunity for self-care when your child or charge is occupied with something else. If they have a favorite television show, you can schedule 30 minutes to dedicate to self-care while they watch TV. Planning ahead is a necessity when caring for someone with ASD, and you need to make sure you don't forget about yourself in the process. Making small changes like these can go a long way in helping you cope with the stress of your role.

Plan Ahead

Take a few minutes before going to bed or after you get up to plan out your day. Make a list of what you want to accomplish and work toward it. Don't forget to schedule in some breaks for self-care. Using a bit of time to prepare for the day to come can save you a lot of worry, chaos, and mistakes. Even if things don't pan out exactly according to plan, having a rough idea of what you need to work toward will avoid wasting time on trying to figure out what you need to do next while you're in the midst of caring for someone else.

Exercise

Physical activities like exercise or taking a walk are great ways to de-stress and maintain your physical health at the same time. Go to the gym or jog around the block, taking a breather away from your child, providing some much-needed respite. You can go alone or with a friend, family member, or neighbor. Taking your pet for a stroll or swimming laps in a pool are some other great ways for a bit of "you time."

Exercise is good for your physical health, improving your mental well-being and relieving stress. It releases endorphins, which have mood-boosting effects to help you feel better mentally and physically. Your sleep quality can improve, which is important because good sleep is essential for overall health. Exercise also helps increase energy levels which is helpful when caring for someone with autism, as the condition can be draining.

Regular physical activity can improve cognitive function and help with decision-making, planning, and problem-solving skills. It's good for your brain since it keeps it awake, stimulated, and relaxed. Supplement your workout regimen with shorter physical activities you can do anywhere and at any time. If you're waiting on water to boil while making dinner, do a few dozen jumping jacks or jog in place. Live in the moment and appreciate every ounce of goodness that comes your way. Finding the time to exercise when you have a child with autism is generally challenging, but even a 30-minute walk each day will make a big difference.

It can be helpful to exercise with a friend or family member to stay motivated. Suppose you don't have time for a formal workout. In that case, there are plenty of alternate ways to fit some exercise into your daily routine, like taking the stairs instead of the elevator or parking further away from your destination.

Take a Bath

Put on your nicest, comfortable house clothes, light scented candles, and take a bath. Place yourself in front of the candles and gaze into the flames. Allow your thoughts to enter your subconscious. Imagine yourself living in a pleasant moment with your child or any beautiful event you wish. See how lovely life is when you fulfill your ambition; this will redirect your attention away from what is going on around you and toward what makes you happy. Following this routine, positive energy runs through you, allowing you to better care for your child.

A hot bath with essential oils and candles is an excellent way to engage your senses and help you relax. The warmth of the water will ease muscle tension, while the oils' scents help calm your mind. The flickering flames of the candles focus your attention and create a sense of peace. Taking some time for yourself in a hot bath with essential oils can make a big difference in your ability to cope with the challenges of caring for someone with autism.

Focus On Positivity

It's tough being a caregiver. Not only do you have to deal with the challenges of caring for someone with a disability, you also have to deal with the constant worry about preventing possible problems from arising for one reason or another. It is easy to get caught up in all of the negative aspects of ASD, but it's important to remember there is also plenty of good in your life. One way to help you cope with this is to focus on positivity. That doesn't mean you have to ignore the challenges of autism, but it does mean focusing on the positive things in your life. When you take the time to focus on the good, it helps you better cope with the bad. So, take a deep breath, relax, and focus on the positive things in your life. You might be surprised at how much better you feel.

Positive Thinking

Think about what would make you happy. Set your mind on something you want to achieve in your life and think about what it will be like when you do. This meditation should focus on positive thoughts and feelings, so the goal doesn't get ruined. Let your mind run wild with this, unlock many possibilities and picture yourself at that moment. You'll notice energy indicating where your mind went when you're finished.

Intentional Thinking

The goal is to get you to think about something other than taking care of a child with autism. Taking your mind off something is a superpower that can help you change your mood. When you feel tired, quickly take your mind on a trip to a new and exciting place.

It could be a sweet memory of something that happened in the past. You will live in that moment for a short time and feel the excitement that comes with it. When you think about good memories, you'll feel more positive and happier. In this enlightened mood, anxiety can't exist, so always keep a positive attitude. You can think deeply and purposefully by making a list of everything you need to make dinner for your family. Use the break to figure out what you need to make that tasty meal. Make this as easy as you can.

Seek Out Professional Help

You have probably read or heard about the many benefits of engaging professional help when you struggle to cope with stress. But what precisely is professional help, and how can it benefit parents and caregivers? Professional help can take many forms, but essentially it is any form of support provided by a trained professional. It includes therapy, counseling, or simply speaking with someone who understands what you are going through.

Engaging professional help can offer a number of benefits for autistic parents and caregivers. It provides a much-needed sounding board for venting about the challenges of raising a child with autism. It can also offer practical advice and support for dealing with difficult behaviors. Perhaps most importantly, it provides a sense of community and connection for those who feel isolated in their experiences. If you are struggling to cope with stress, engaging professional help might be the best decision you ever make.

What Next?

Finding enough time to care for yourself is challenging when caring for a child with special needs. Decide on at least one self-care activity every day, whether 5 minutes of mindfulness meditation before you get out of bed or 10 minutes of squats. Then, aim to implement more and more as time goes on.

Whatever self-care routine you choose, remember, as long as you're doing something that benefits you in the present, you will be making a giant leap toward a more balanced daily life that will benefit everyone involved. But, most importantly, you.

CHAPTER EIGHT

ACTIVITIES FOR YOURSELF AND TOGETHER

As a caregiver, you won't always be able to carve out 30-60 minutes for yourself while looking after the needs of others. It's easy to become so preoccupied with your responsibilities that you forget about yourself entirely. There will be times when your charge requires too much attention to take a long bath or walk around the block. However, studies have shown that even very brief breaks have a significant effect on helping people cope with stress. There are plenty of self-care options that can be done in only five minutes, and you can do them no matter where you are.

Five Minute Self-Care Ideas

Practice Breathing Exercises

Using breathing exercises as a sort of "mini-meditation" can allow you to perform some self-care no matter what else you happen to be doing at the moment. You can do them while cooking, cleaning, driving around, doing chores, or even just sitting down and relaxing.

Keeping your mouth closed, slowly inhale through your nostrils while counting to 4. Hold the air in your lungs and count to 7. Then exhale slowly through your mouth, while counting to 8. This is known as "4-7-8 Breathing."

You can use this tactic as frequently as you can, particularly if your child is prone to throwing temper tantrums. Just give yourself a few moments to stop, and breathe. Find a few moments of peace and quiet so that you can take a few deep breaths and collect your thoughts.

Play on Your Phone

Set aside 5 minutes every few hours to just fiddle around mindlessly on your phone. Go ahead and scroll through TikTok, browse Instagram, or reply to people on Facebook. Taking short breaks to consume social media can actually help you feel better. People are social creatures, and through social media, you can connect with others even when you can't physically meet with them.

You can also bring up a site like YouTube and watch a video or two. Comedy videos can be particularly beneficial, as they will undoubtedly make you laugh. Laughter helps shift your energy and ease stress, so laugh out loud if possible. Create a library of amusing clips to access anytime you take your 5 minute break.

Playing certain mobile games can also work during these brief windows of opportunity. You can't delve into a more involved game, but something like Candy Crush or crossword puzzles that let you complete one level and then save more for later are generally the best types of games to use for 5 minute self-care.

Have a Cup of Tea or Coffee

Enjoying a cup of coffee or tea can be very enjoyable, especially when you can get a 5 minute break during the day. You can drink something with caffeine, which provides you with a boost of energy. Even if you prefer decaf, people just find the flavor and experience of drinking a warm beverage to be relaxing and soothing.

Listen to Music

Listening to music is one of the simplest activities you can do for self-care, as you can do it while performing just about any other task. Most songs don't last more than 3 or 4 minutes, and if you have earbuds, you can listen as you take care of your responsibilities. Research has shown that music helps reduce stress, boost moods, and improve overall well-being. Anything that can help reduce stress is a good thing.

Listening to music is a great way to motivate you or unwind after a long day. It also helps you relax and fall asleep more easily. If you're feeling stressed or anxious, music calms you down. There are even specific music genres specifically helpful for people with autism. So, whether you're looking to relax or boost your mood, there's music out there that can help.

Furthermore, listening to music isn't merely about finding something that sounds good. It's also about finding something that resonates with you personally. So, don't be afraid to experiment until you find the right mix of artists and genres that work for you. Remember, when taking care of yourself, there's no one-size-fits-all solution.

Take a Power Shower

Power showers aren't like typical showers, where the goal is to clean all the dirt and oils from your hair and skin. They are meant to be a jolt to your system, essentially "rebooting" your body and mind about halfway through the day. The key to successful power showers is cold water. If you try it with hot or tepid water, it won't provide the shock to your central nervous system that makes it effective.

A quick, cold shower doesn't just wake you up in the same way as having an ice bucket tossed over your head. It can improve the circulation of your blood and reduce muscle soreness, which is great if you've been engaging in physical activity all day. When you get in the shower, remain beneath the water for as long as you can manage. Don't overdo it, though—2 or 3 minutes maximum is more than enough. By the time you dry off and get dressed again, only about 5 minutes will have passed, and you'll be ready to tackle any challenges that come your way.

Activities You Can Do for You

Of course, your activities don't have to be for only 5 minutes. It's important to take of yourself in other ways so you don't feel like you're burning out. Here are a few tips

Ask for Help

When you've had enough, don't be afraid to speak up. You can get help from a family member, friend, or co-worker. You might employ assistance on days when you need to take a break and rest.

There is no medal for the most stressed person on the planet, so reach out to someone right away to help you. As a parent or caregiver to a neurodiversity child, you might believe that no one can provide the same level of care you provide. You're mistaken. Doing things on your own will exhaust you.

Listen to Your Best Music

The sound of music can help you feel better in an instant. Choose your favorite music so you can have a good time. Within 5 minutes, you can listen to one or two tracks. There is a saying that "music is life," and it has the ability to revive your spirit.

Dance

Dancing has a way of lifting anyone's spirits. Make some legendary moves while listening to your favorite songs. Don't be shy; you're the only one in the room. Who knows, it could also be fun for the autistic child, but you're dancing to make yourself happy first. Dancing should be entertaining.

Try Yoga Pose

One of the best activities available to reduce stress is yoga. Bring out your yoga mat, dust it off, and try some poses. Afterward, you will feel much better. You will also progressively speed up feeling better by stretching your joints.

Delegate Some Work

You are not a horse; therefore, don't try to work like one. If necessary, delegate some of your workload to someone else, like your spouse or a family member. You need all the spare time you can get, so seize the opportunity when it presents itself. Go outside for 5 minutes to obtain some fresh air before returning to your chores.

Create "Me" Time

When caring for your children, especially those with autism, it is normal to get so preoccupied that you give up on your goals, hobbies, leisure time, and even getting a decent day or night's rest. You must have a time and day set aside to do the things you enjoy. Go for a spa treatment, pedicure, manicure, or anything within your grasp.

This day is all about you; do things that make you happy and feel better. Utilize these days to rest, eat, sleep, or watch your favorite movie. It is critical that you keep your identity outside of caring for a neurodivergent child. Use your "me time" to accomplish activities that are simple but rejuvenating. If time does not allow for a lengthy break, make it basic and brief.

Hug a Loved One

Reaching out for a quick hug from your partner if they are nearby can alleviate stress and bring you back to a calm state of mind. Whether it's a family member or a friend, you're free to hug them. After completing this exercise, expect your adrenaline to start pumping.

Show Yourself Some Love

You already know what you enjoy and what you can do to make yourself feel special. It could be taking a few minutes to order your favorite meal or drink. While you wait for it to arrive, the anticipation of how sweet and yummy. The food will keep you excited and bubbling. The state of your mind, body, and heart as an autistic child caretaker will decide how effective your caregiving can be. Putting your health first means providing the best care possible.

Massage

If your partner is nearby, that's great, but if not, go for a quick neck massage. You will also feel better quickly by massaging your feet and hands with essential oil. Massage is good for you and can be used to relieve stress quickly and stimulate sensory organs.

Documentation

Taking a few minutes away from your work to document your experience will make you feel better. Writing about your path as a caregiver allows you to realize how many fights you have won and how far you have come. You will undoubtedly receive some praise for your efforts, and this alone will improve your mood.

A Quick Bath

Many people go to the bathroom to relax their bodies and lift their spirits. A quick shower in cold water can help you calm down. While you shower, a few drops of essential oil in the tub will make you feel much better. For the ladies, a quick hair wash goes a long way toward making you feel better.

Have a List of Gratitude

There should be many things for which you are grateful, now is the time to write them down. As you note your gratitude, your energy shifts and radiates with positivity. You will realize how much you have accomplished and how many advantages you have taken for granted. Make this list whenever you start to feel like a loser; it serves as a fast reminder that heals.

Wash Your Face

A quick face wash face might be soothing when you're feeling worried. When caring for a neurodiversity child becomes stressful and your anxiety level rises, quickly wash your face, and return to your activity. The use of soap is not necessary for the effectiveness of this exercise; water will do.

Drink Water

Yes, a glass of water while you sit and mind your own business will help you feel better. Concentrate only on the water. Read the label on the water bottle and purposefully admire the container to maintain your focus. The goal is to distract and calm your mind.

Make a To-Do List

Take five minutes to make a list of everything you wish to do. It might be countries you'd like to visit, the food you'd like to try someday, your happiest memories, favorite television shows, happiest excursion with a buddy or spouse, and so on. The list should only include positive items. Your energy level must be at an all-time high to work well as an autistic child caregiver. For the best outcomes, your mental state should be stable.

Tend to Your Pet

Pets are affectionate animals who will willingly yield to being petted. Pets give off a warm and fuzzy vibe. A little downtime with your pet, perhaps just sitting and caressing them, helps to slow your heartbeat and relax you.

Compliment Yourself

Make a list of all the amazing things about yourself. Continue writing for as long as the list lasts until the 5 minutes are over. When caring for an autistic child, you usually lose yourself and devote all your focus to the child. It appears like you are no longer living, so take a few moments to remind yourself how amazing you are. You will feel better as a result.

Practice Positive Affirmation

Tell yourself positive things. Tell yourself you are loved, and everything is going well for you. Tell yourself that the universe knows how hard things are, and you will always have the resources and energy to keep going until the end of time. Assure yourself that money won't be a problem because people will come to your aid. These affirmations are like a law for your life; if you believe them, you will get what they say.

Do Backward Counting

It is simple to count up without paying attention and make few or no mistakes. You have to pay attention when you count backward, and it's a way to meditate. Before you can say a number, you must be able to see it; this will help you get back to being calm.

Check Up on Friends

It's always nice to spend time with friends. You and your friends can get on a conference call to talk about things that have nothing to do with autism. Checking up on someone makes you feel like you matter to them and gives you peace of mind that they are doing well. It will make you feel better.

Take a Deep Breath

You can ease your anxiety and relax by giving yourself a series of five deep breaths in a row. Perform this activity several times to get your energy level back under control. Following this, you will feel energy and positivity.

Check Up on Your Garden

A simple walk around your garden to check your fauna and flora's progress is beneficial for a mental shift. Water the garden and admire the lovely sight of green vegetables. Seeing how nicely your garden is doing will give you confidence that you are capable of great things. Bring a few fresh flowers from your garden inside to brighten the space and give it a natural sense.

Gist Time with Your Spouse

A pep chat with your partner can be beneficial. A few

minutes of discussion with them can lift your spirits. If they are around, have them sit while you rest your head on their lap. While the talk is going on, a gentle hair stroke from your partner will help you relax faster.

Read a Cook Book

Read for five minutes and discover something new to add to your culinary repertoire; this is the equivalent of slaying two birds with one stone. While reading the book takes your mind off your autistic caregiving experiences, it also teaches you new things to include in your cuisine to create a beautiful dinner. Make a list of the recipes you'd like to try while reading.

Let Some Sunlight into the Room

The sensation of sunlight on your face as you wake up in the morning is transformative. It instantly energizes and gets you ready to start your day. Make it a habit to open the windows as soon as you wake up to let in fresh air and sunlight. It will immediately change the energy in the room. A few minutes of action can set the tone for the rest of your day.

Activities You Can Do as a Caregiver

While self-care that focuses solely on yourself is important, sometimes engaging in a fun activity with the person you're caring for can offer benefits for you and your charges. People with ASD need to socialize and be entertained just like anyone else. Doing something together kills two birds with one stone, as you'll still be taking care of them, but in a way that is less stressful than if you were just sitting around the house.

Tips for Finding the Right Activities

Choose an Activity You Both Enjoy

Finding ways to get an individual with ASD to engage in simple activities or perform tasks as part of a daily routine isn't always easy, especially if it's something they don't want to do. Many parents, caregivers, and educators will come up with creative methods of catching and holding the attention of someone with ASD. You can turn it into a game or a contest, making it seem like fun. You can get ideas for what to do from just about anywhere, as long as you keep an open mind.

While you and those you're caring for may have different interests, it can be immensely gratifying to find an activity you both enjoy. If you are not sure what they like, try asking them about their favorite characters, shows, or games. Children with ASD tend to have a lot of energy and are constantly wanting to move their bodies, so physical activities that allow them to burn off that energy are a good choice. They are also good visual learners, so activities involving pictures or symbols will be helpful. Most often, you will find them more interested in nonverbal activities.

Make it Short and Sweet

Remember, people with ASD often have shorter attention spans than someone that is neurotypical. So, when you plan an activity, make sure to keep it short and sweet. Allowing something to go on too long runs the risk of becoming boring to them, and they may begin to act up if they don't feel like they're getting the right kind of stimulation. Choose an activity you can do in a short amount of time, like 15-30 minutes.

Be Flexible

Be prepared to change the activity if it is not working. If the person you're caring for isn't interested in the activity or is getting frustrated, try something else. It is important to be flexible and adjust what you're doing on the fly. Sometimes, individuals with ASD will have their own way of playing a game that doesn't follow the standard rules. Letting them teach you how they like to perform an activity and going along with it can make them feel more confident about similar interactions in the future.

Make It Part of the Routine

Making activities a part of your daily routine helps make them more enjoyable for both of you. Pick a convenient time for when you can both do the activity at the same time each day.

Activity Ideas

There are many different activities you can do with your autistic child. Here are a few ideas:

Arts and Crafts

Arts and crafts are a great way to spend time together and can be very therapeutic. You can do many different projects, such as painting, sculpting, or making collages. If you are unsure where to start, many books and websites offer ideas and instructions.

Music

Listening to music or playing instruments is a great way to relax and is very calming for children with autism. You can play music together or listen to it while doing other activities.

Sports

Playing sports is a great way to get both of you moving. You can play catch, shoot hoops, or go for a swim. Doing something active together is a great way to relieve stress and have fun.

Games

Playing games is another great way to spend time together and can be very stimulating for children with autism. Available in various avenues are many different games you can play, such as board games, card games, or video games.

You can also make up your games.

Reading to Them

Reading aloud to someone with ASD is a great way to stimulate their mind and help them learn. It can also be very calming. Choose books that are interesting to your child, and make sure to read with expression. Also, look at the pictures together and talk about the stories.

Nature

Spending time in nature is a great way to relax and can be very calming for children with autism. You can go for a walk, hike, or bike ride. You can also look for birds or other animals. Even a simple stroll around the block can be beneficial. If you are unsure where to go, many websites and books offer ideas.

Cooking

Cooking is an excellent way to spend time together and can be very therapeutic. You will never be short of the many recipes you can try, such as simple snacks or meals. You can also bake cookies or cakes together. Also, you can try recipes that do not require cooking, such as fruit salads or smoothies.

Dancing

Dancing is a great way to get both of you moving and can be very stimulating. You can dance to music together or make up your own dances.

Whatever you choose, make sure you are having fun and enjoying yourselves. Spending time together is the most important thing. Don't forget to reward your child afterward.

These are some self-care tips for adults who care for children with autism. Making time for yourself can be difficult, but finding ways to reduce your stress is important.

Taking care of yourself is important for everyone, but it is exceptionally significant for caregivers. When you take care of yourself, you can better care for the people who depend on you. Self-care is not selfish. It is a necessary part of caring for others. Make sure to take the time to care for yourself physically and emotionally.

CHAPTER NINE

SUPPORTING A CAREGIVER

Even if you aren't personally a caregiver, there are things you can do to support those in your life that are. It's a complicated and exhausting role, but it's also necessary, as individuals with ASD often aren't able to be self-sufficient, even after they've reached adulthood. Caring for them can be a lifelong commitment, and some caregivers will remain the primary caregiver for the majority of the person's life. Not everyone is capable of making the kinds of sacrifices necessary to be a caregiver, but that doesn't mean you can't help them out in some way.

Educating Others

Take a moment to think about what autism looks like. It's estimated that 1 in 54 children in the U.S. has autism, making it one of the most common developmental disorders. Now, try to imagine what it feels like to not just live with autism, but be the parent or caregiver of someone with autism. It's not an easy task, and with so much time being dedicated to their children, it doesn't leave them many opportunities to sit down with others and help guide them through what their life is like.

Parents and caregivers will naturally be very well-versed in the facts and realities surrounding ASD, but the bulk of their attention needs to remain on the people they're caring for. However, it's also important to educate those around you about the condition, especially if they will be having any sort of relationship or communications with the child. ASD can be an isolating experience, but by learning as much as possible about it, you can help a caregiver build a support network of understanding people.

By taking on the task of educating others about ASD, you're removing the entirety of the burden from the caregiver, which can often be a great relief. There will still be aspects of ASD that only a parent or caregiver can or should explain, but as far as the basics of autism and how it affects people, that is something you can easily teach them. In addition, keeping friends and family informed about how autism affects one's day-to-day life can go a long way toward easing any stress and tension that might arise over misunderstandings or miscommunication.

Tips for Educating Others about Autism

1. **Start with the basics.** Explain what autism is and how it affects behavior and social interaction.

2. **Be open about your experiences.** Share stories about your child's challenges and successes.

3. **Be patient.** It might take time for others to understand and accept your child's diagnosis.

4. **Seek out resources.** Many great books, websites, and support groups are available to help people learn more about autism.

By taking the time to educate those around you about autism, you can help create a more supportive and understanding environment for yourself and your loved ones. Many problems that crop up when non-caregivers deal with individuals with ASD only occur due to the person being misinformed or ignorant about autism. Understanding breeds connection, and it's much likelier that someone will be patient and work within the parameters of a person with ASD's comfort zone.

Ways to Help a Caregiver

Pack a Bag for Them

As a parent of an autistic child, you should grasp the need for consistency and planning. Why not schedule some time for yourself as part of your preparation? Prepare a bag so you don't have to search the house for the things you'll need to exit the front door. Make sure you have enough space in your bag pack for a few additional items to keep you amused during any unplanned downtime.

These items could be a book or magazine, athletic equipment, crocheting, gardening gloves, or even a pair of headphones - whatever it is, it should be something you can pick up and start doing right away. But don't overpack. The key to a good trip is to focus on the essentials. You don't want your bag to become a burden.

Practice Mindfulness

You can help a caregiver by being aware of what challenges they're facing, and what help they could use to make their workload a bit lighter. Mindfulness can help break the cycle of stress and anxiety. It's about being present in the moment and doing what you can to improve the situation without trying to control everything. Helping a caregiver in this way will aid them in coping with the challenges of their job.

Optimism and Emotional Acceptance

Cultivating optimism in a caregiver brings a sense of positivity to their role. A positive outlook can improve a person's mood and alleviate anxiety, so helping a caregiver see the good in a situation may benefit them when they're struggling. It's also been linked to better health outcomes, so it's worth making an effort to cultivate optimism in their life and your own.

Another helpful coping strategy is encouraging emotional acceptance, meaning accepting one's emotions for what they are, and not fighting them or pushing them away. It isn't easy, but it's an important step in managing stress. If the caregiver can accept their emotions when feeling upset, tired, or frustrated, they'll be in a better position to do their job.

Offer Assistance with Chores

People are sometimes afraid to ask for help when they need it, as it makes them feel like they've failed and will reflect poorly upon them. When someone is responsible for caring for an individual with ASD, they may also not want to burden anyone else with their problems, so they'll avoid telling their support system when they're overwhelmed.

Offering to lend them a hand with their responsibilities when you can often does more for them than you might think. Picking up the dry cleaning, doing the dishes, or doing a bit of grocery shopping may seem like small favors to you, but when a caregiver is dealing with someone with ASD, even the little things start to add up, increasing the burden on their shoulders. Having even a tiny bit of that weight taken off them can make a huge difference for caregivers.

Be Reassuring

When someone is already overwhelmed by the enormity of their responsibilities, even a small mistake can feel like a major crisis. When you see a caregiver in this kind of headspace, try to reassure them that it's not as big a deal as they thought. They might spill a glass of coffee on your shirt and become despondent, beating themselves up over it because of the pressure they're under. Just tell them, "It's not a big deal. I can easily change my clothing quickly."

Consider what you'd say to a good friend if your child were experiencing a full-fledged meltdown at the mall, on a public bus, or any of the other horrible public places where you'd be stuck alone with a fuming child. For example, "I'm sure you'll pull through. You're a hero." It requires attentiveness and a lot of work, so if you make a mistake, talk to yourself like a good friend.

Recognize Their Accomplishments

When the day is over, people often think about all the things they couldn't accomplish. On the other hand, they rarely congratulate themselves for doing something well. Find something that a caregiver did during that day and give them a compliment about it. Tell them how proud you are of them, and that you see how hard they work all the time. You will be shocked when you see how much of a difference this can make in their demeanor. It gives them the confidence to begin the process all over again the next day.

Talk to Friends and Family

Naturally, the people a caregiver trusts more will be their close friends and family members. Do not hesitate to speak with them whenever you see a caregiver becoming overwhelmed. Depending on their time, they can assist you in many ways. Some will listen and talk them through stressful situations, while others will help with the usual tasks and responsibilities. Either way, nobody has to go through everything by themselves.

It always pays off to be open about your struggles to the people you trust and ask for their help. Some will even volunteer to spend time with your child or ask you to bring your child when you visit. Never perceive this as a bad thing. Besides those you meet with regularly, there are other people you will probably never see in your entire life but who can be very helpful and supportive.

Massage Therapy

As an autism caregiver, you know that the job is rewarding and challenging. One of the biggest challenges is managing stress. Fortunately, massage therapy is a great way to help relieve stress and improve your well-being. Massage therapy increases circulation promotes relaxation and reduces muscle tension. When you receive a message, your body releases endorphins, which are natural painkillers that boost your mood and ease anxiety. In addition, massage therapy increases flexibility and range of motion, which is helpful when caring for someone with autism. Receiving regular massages will make you feel more relaxed and better able to handle the challenges of caregiving. If you're interested in massage therapy, be sure to speak with your doctor or a certified massage therapist to find out more.

Encourage Communication

There is nothing wrong with seeking psychological assistance, whether through individual treatment, support groups, mentorship, or online counseling. Anyone in need of aid can get it. You might find some extremely beneficial information if you research counseling support suggestions. The primary goal is to encourage a caregiver to communicate their thoughts, feelings, concerns, and fears with somebody willing to listen.

Sometimes, parents may find it difficult adjusting to a new diagnosis, learning new parenting skills or about events, learning stress-management techniques, and embracing new ways to stay connected with their partners and life activities. Make sure you always let them know that you'll be happy to lend them an ear. Sometimes, all they will need is to vocalize something that's been eating away at them, and once they hear it out loud, they can see their worries were unfounded.

Remind Them to Have Fun

We all have many things we enjoy doing. You will appreciate life a lot more by giving yourself time to do the things you love and meeting people whose company you enjoy. Having fun will immediately result in happiness, which helps you cope better with every aspect of life.

Life is much more than just hard work and struggle. Even if taking care of your child takes most of your time and energy, allow yourself some pleasant activities and release the pressure and stress that come with your everyday tasks and responsibilities.

Again, you can choose to have fun on your own or with others, as both are very rewarding. Doing fun stuff alone is a good indication that you appreciate yourself and can enjoy your own company. Sharing that with others, whether your partner, family, or friends, will help you bond more and create wonderful memories that will last for a lifetime.

CHAPTER TEN

FINDING THE RIGHT BALANCE BETWEEN CAREGIVING AND SELF-CARE

One of the trickiest aspects of being a successful caregiver is finding the right balance between your responsibilities to the individual with ASD and your duty to keep yourself healthy. If you don't spend enough time on self-care, your health and ability to care for your charge can suffer, but spending too much time on yourself may result in neglecting the person you're meant to help. It is important to have a plan in place that gives you enough time to yourself to avoid burnout, while still satisfying all the needs a person with ASD requires.

Get Enough Sleep

Sleep is essential for everyone, but getting enough is crucial for caregivers of people with ASD. When well-rested, you will have more patience and energy to deal with challenging behaviors. Sleep recharges and reboots your brain in preparation for the new day. Make time for a decent, peaceful sleep no matter how busy you are—

preferably 6-8 hours.

Our decision-making abilities and stress management tools can be severely affected by exhaustion. So, make it a must to get at least four hours of sleep every day, and if you can afford to increase the sleeping time, please do so. Try taking naps when your child does, syncing your sleeping patterns so you can have more reliable opportunities to remain well-rested.

People with ASD may have difficulties going to sleep and sleeping through the night, so if they keep waking up in need of assistance, you won't be getting enough sleep, either.. Try to establish a bedtime routine for them, creating a calming environment, and avoid allowing them any stimulants before going to sleep. Some stimulants that keep you up at night include caffeine, nicotine, and certain medications. If they are taking medication for ASD or autism-related symptoms, talk to their doctor about potential side effects that could be interfering with their ability to sleep at night.

Eat Healthy Foods

Eating a healthy diet is important for everyone, but it is especially crucial for people caring for individuals with ASD. You may already spend a significant amount of time and effort preparing nutritious meals for those under your care, yet you will settle for something less healthy for yourself. There is certainly a tradeoff, as when you're very busy, you may simply not have enough time to feed yourself and others. However, you should do your best to avoid reaching for junk food or unhealthy snacks. They will only make you feel worse in the long run.

The best option when you are running on a tight schedule is to have a healthy snack, like fruit or mixed nuts, until you've taken care of your duties. Once you have some free time, possibly after others have gone to bed, you can make yourself a proper meal. If you get up before anyone else, you can make a balanced breakfast. Having nutritious food to maintain your energy levels and remain fit can allow you to do more with your day.

Focus on eating plenty of fresh fruits and vegetables, whole grains, lean protein, and healthy fats. Avoid processed foods and sugary snacks as much as possible. It will also help you stay hydrated by drinking plenty of water throughout the day.Certain foods have been known to be beneficial for people with ASD, such as omega-3 fatty acids, vitamin B6, vitamin C, magnesium, and probiotics. These nutrients help improve mood, reduce anxiety, and promote a healthy gut. Adding these superfoods to your diet will improve everyone's health.

When you know you're going to be particularly busy in the days ahead, set aside some time to make some recipes in bulk. You can cook enough breakfasts, lunches, and dinners for the upcoming week, storing them in the freezer. Once mealtime comes around, all you'll need to do is retrieve the portions and heat them up. Eating at the same time every day might also assist in providing structure to your life. You'll see the benefits almost immediately.

Journaling

One of the best ways to manage the stress of caregiving is to keep a journal. If you're struggling with depression, stress, or anxiety, and find it challenging to communicate your suffering, then getting it all out on paper can help you understand the roots of these issues. You might discover thoughts and feelings you never considered an issue or find things that trigger you by identifying common thought patterns.

Journaling gives you a chance to vent all your frustrations in a private and safe setting. It can be a huge relief, especially if you're overwhelmed. It will aid you in organizing your thoughts and making sense of what's happening in your life. In addition, journaling assists you in making sense of your emotions and finding ways to cope with the caregiving challenges.

Journaling is also a great way to track your progress. As you reflect on your entries, you'll see how far you've come and the challenges you've overcome. You can track your loved one's progress and celebrate their accomplishments. It can be incredibly motivating, helping you move forward, even when things are tough.

Keeping a journal can help you to connect with other caregivers. You can find many online communities where people share their experiences, offering support to one another. In these communities, you'll find people who understand what you're going through and offer valuable advice and perspective.

Writing in a journal can be a great way to express your thoughts and feelings. You can witness your progress by keeping a journal, allowing you to track your daily routine and which goals you've been able to accomplish. There are no rules for journal writing, so you can write about whatever you like. You will find it helpful to write about your day-to-day experiences, hopes, and fears for the future.

Another great way is to keep a gratitude journal, where you write down things you are thankful for each day. Making a gratitude list helps shift your focus from negative to positive thoughts.

You can also record your child's milestones in a journal or write about the challenges you are facing. Journal writing is an excellent way to offload some of your worries and help you see things from a different perspective.

This is another kind of self-care that parents of autistic children may employ. In a variety of ways, journaling can help you improve your mental health. It allows parents to recover from daily stressors and leave the unimportant stuff behind; it allows them to express all of their emotions on paper, reducing stress and tension. It improves their overall sense of well-being and gratitude while reducing depression symptoms, intrusion, and knock-off symptoms of post-trauma, improving their working memory, and boosting their mood.

Reduce the Distractions

As a result of technology improvements, disruptive sounds and demands have entered your life. You could find yourself checking your phone to take a break from your day, but you are unaware you are stressing yourself further. You look at the lives of others on social media and think, "Wow, I can't imagine how that would appear on me?" Alternatively, you feel additional waves of anxiety due to reading the news.

The truth is that when you don't let negative and damaging disruptions into your environment, it becomes much easier to handle. That tiny device in your hand has the potential to cause havoc. So, take a break from electronics to reduce distractions, including putting the phone down and, if possible, turning it off for a few minutes.

Breaking away from your daily struggles and spending time alone, without any distractions, can positively affect your mental health. Finding time to be alone can be challenging at first, but start with as little as 10 or 15 minutes every day. The time you spend alone, especially at night, will help you contemplate and gather your thoughts and feelings without the pressure and many distractions of busier times during the day. You will be much more clear-minded and easily wrap your head around complicated issues. You will also learn to appreciate yourself more and gain a deeper and better understanding of who you are.

Spending time alone is also an excellent way to slow down and recharge. You will most certainly feel better afterward and regain the much-needed energy to keep going. In addition, allow your mind to wander and get lost in your imagination. The sense of freedom of being lost in your imagination will improve your mental health and boost your creativity, helping you become more productive in everything you do.

Exercise Regularly

Getting regular exercise is important for physical and mental health. It reduces stress, improves mood, and increases energy levels. As a caregiver, you might not have much time for exercise. Figuring out the best way to fit it into your schedule can prevent you from falling behind on your healthcare goals. It's always easier to exercise when you do it every day or every few days for 15-45 minutes, rather than wait until you have a block of time free to work out for a couple of hours.

Tips for Getting Regular Exercise

- **Walk or Bike:** One of the easiest ways to integrate regular exercise into your routine is to walk or ride a bike when you need to go somewhere. As long as you don't need to go too far, choosing one of these options over driving in a car will let you get a bit of a workout, while at the same time completing whatever tasks you have to get done.

- **Join an Exercise Class:** Exercise classes are a great way to get regular exercise. Many different exercise classes are available, so you can find one that is right for you.

- **Use Exercise Equipment at Home:** If you have exercise equipment at home, like a treadmill or elliptical machine, you can use it to workout when you have some free time. You don't even need machines like something you'd find at the gym— pull up bars, jump ropes, and free weights are all small, easily moved pieces of equipment that you can use to ensure you can exercise while fitting it into your schedule.

- **Play Games and Activities:** You can play games or do activities that require physical exertion.

There are a plethora of ideas you can try, such as tag or hide-and-seek. Shooting hoops, throwing around a ball, or foot races are also enjoyable activities you can partake in, especially with younger children.

- **Get Your Others Involved:** Try making plans for physical activity involving other people, like a partner, family member, friend, or neighbor. This is a great way to get both of you moving, and having someone else to help motivate you can keep you from neglecting your exercises.

Make Time for Yourself

It is essential to make time for yourself, even if it is only a few minutes each day. It helps you reduce stress and feel more relaxed. As a parent or caregiver of a child with autism, you might feel you do not have time for yourself. However, finding ways to make time for your needs is important.

Tips for Making Time for Yourself

Set Aside Time Each Day

Set aside at least 30 minutes each day for yourself. During this time, you can do something that you enjoy, such as reading, listening to music, or taking a bath. You can do anything that will help you relax and feel good.

You can do many crafts, projects, or whatever you like as long as it is something that makes you feel good.

Take Breaks

Taking breaks throughout the day will reduce stress and refresh you. If possible, take a break when your child takes a break; this can help you have some time to yourself.

Ask for Help

Asking for help from family and friends is a great way to reduce stress. You may feel you have to do everything yourself, but this is not the case. You might feel pressured to go above and beyond, overworking yourself to care for a child or charge with ASD. But parents are not obligated to devote their entire selves to their children. It's fine to seek assistance from time to time, or even every day if necessary. Asking for help allows you to have more time for yourself.

Regardless of your thoughts or feelings, you should know when to seek and get support. Parents don't always require child care assistance, but they could require aid with home duties. For example, hire a lawn service to mow the grass and water the plants in the garden, or ask friends to prepare a few meals for you. As a parent of a special needs child, the more assistance you can obtain, the more time you will have for yourself and your children. Do not hesitate to ask for help when you feel yourself reaching your limits. There's nothing to be ashamed about if you need a breather.

Schedule Time for Yourself

Schedule time for yourself each week, as you would schedule time for doctor's appointments or grocery shopping. It will help ensure that you actually make time for yourself. Even if you schedule a half hour of listening to music or playing a game, actually having it on the agenda means you're less likely to skip it in favor of doing more work.

Find a Babysitter

If you have trouble finding time for yourself, consider hiring a babysitter, giving you some time each week to do something you enjoy without worrying about your child. Depending on the severity of your child's ASD, you may need to pay a little more to get someone experienced in caring for people with autism.

Respite Care

If you don't have a family member or friend who can babysit, seek respite care in your area to help you recharge and focus on yourself, even if it's only for a few hours a week. Respite care is temporary care provided by someone else for your child with ASD. It can allow you a much-needed break from the demands of caring for a child with ASD, and you focus on other aspects of your life, such as your job or relationship. Your relationships will suffer if you do not take care of yourself. If there is a family emergency, having a good relationship with one respite provider gives you a trusted caregiver for your child. Respite care allows you to unwind and relax while also avoiding stress and tiredness.

Join a Support Group

Joining a support group for caregivers of those with special needs can be extremely beneficial. Parenting a child with ASD is often isolating, so seeking out support from others in a similar situation is important. Many online and local support groups are available for parents of children with ASD. Talking to parents going through similar experiences is very helpful. You can also talk to your child's doctor or a mental health professional if you struggle to cope.

You can also find support groups meant for caregivers of adults and elderly individuals with ASD. The experience as this type of caregiver has some overlap with parents of children with ASD, but you will largely be focusing on managing different aspects of the disability. An adult does not need to go to school, and their therapies generally target gaps in their abilities instead of education across the board.

You will receive advice, information, and a shoulder to cry on in the support group, especially on difficult days. Being around people going through the same ordeal as you will help you mentally and keep you from isolating yourself or feeling depressed after your child is diagnosed with autism syndrome disorder. Make it a point to schedule and attend meetings in the support group to which you belong. Remember that you must maintain your mental health to deal with the challenges of caring for a child with ASD.

Tips for Finding a Support Group

Ask Your Doctor or Therapist

Your doctor or therapist can recommend a support group in your area. Many different support groups are available, so be sure to ask about the specific group you are looking for. These support groups are provided by a variety of charitable organizations. There are others that you can join online as well. Attending workshops or gatherings can help you meet other members of the community. Your purposeful efforts in caring for your child will be recognized and respected.

Online Forums

The Internet can be absolutely great. Using the appropriate online forums, you can easily and anonymously open up to total strangers and expect them to cheer you up and support you in any way they can. Online forums are full of people with similar experiences and professionals. Both share valuable tips on how to deal with any given situation.

You can content yourself with sharing your thoughts and feelings in these online groups. Many people will support you emotionally by sharing their experiences. Alternatively, if you have specific questions, you can share them and ask for advice. The great thing about online forums is that people who give advice do so genuinely and out of sheer love and compassion; they expect nothing in return.

Making sure your autistic child lives a happy life has probably taken a lot of your time, money, and efforts, as well as your physical and mental health. However, by no means should you let that deplete and bring you down. An ASD child requires extensive care, but so do you. Your well-being and your child's go hand in hand, and you should never neglect either.

We have seen how essential it is to allow your child to do many things and meet other people to help them grow and develop their personality and skills. We have also shown the importance of caring for your physical and mental health, either by spending time alone or sharing moments with your family and close friends.

Despite the difficulties, you will most certainly achieve a lot. Every day does not have to feel like a struggle. Instead, regard each day as another opportunity to learn, grow, and improve, whether for you or your child.

Ask Other Parents

Other parents and caregivers of children with autism can

recommend a support group in your area. People going through the same will also be able to support you. Finding people who are raising a child with ASD like you is thankfully not as difficult these days as it once was. Parents often belong to organizations that allow them to meet others dealing with similar issues, so they are a great resource to use.

It is convenient that the groups meet in the evening, allowing parents to sit and talk about their recent experiences, discuss home strategies that have worked, share what hasn't worked, and get advice from other parents in similar situations. These get-togethers are a great way for parents to take care of themselves while also meeting new people.

Call Your Local Autism Agency

Your local autism agency will help you find a support group in your area. Many national organizations offer support groups for parents and caregivers of children with autism.

Get Involved in Group Activities

You can also get both of you moving by participating in activities. You can play active games together, go for walks, or bike rides. Doing things together will help you feel connected to your child and can be a great way to reduce stress.

Be Social

Socialize with Others

Experience has shown that when caring for someone with autism, caregivers often need to find ways to relieve stress and improve their well-being. Unwinding and heading out with friends are two great ways. When caregivers take a break from their caregiving duties, it gives them a chance to recharge their batteries and return to their responsibilities refreshed and ready to face the challenges ahead. In addition, socializing with friends reduces stress by providing a much-needed outlet for conversation and laughter. Moreover, getting out and about increases caregivers' sense of community and connection, further boosting their mood and overall well-being. So, the next time you're feeling overwhelmed, remember that taking some time out for yourself is good for your body and mind.

Make New Friends

Any child can have a hard time making new friends, especially children with autism. You can never be sure of what the other kids' reactions will be. In particular, you should pay attention to their first experience with a friend and ensure it will not be traumatic. Children with ASD can become friends with other autistic children at their specialized schools just like with other children.

You should definitely help your child develop social skills in as many settings and with as many people as possible. All you must do is allow them the freedom to cope with the different social situations and closely observe how they cope. How they communicate, express their emotions, and deal with the inevitable conflicts will give insight into what to focus on and improve.

Of course, you will not always be around when they're at school. In this case, speak to the school staff and discuss how they will adapt your child's social skills. Accordingly, they can advise on what to do at home to help your child improve their social abilities.

Learn How to Meditate

Meditation is an excellent way to unwind and clear your mind of things you can't change or control. Autism in children can be managed or reduced, but it cannot be cured. Over time, you will notice a major shift in your child's behavior and cognitive functioning.

There is much evidence that regular meditation and mindfulness practices enhance the body's health mentally and physically. Mindfulness and meditation help with anxiety, despair, and chronic pain.

You can set out 15 minutes in the morning before the kids wake up or before you go to bed to listen to something that would improve your mind. As you feel more comfortable with meditation, increase how many minutes you spend on it. Parents use many free apps to start their meditation practice wherever they are.

These are excellent approaches that autistic parents should employ. Rather than allowing yourself to wallow in sadness, meditation will assist in focusing on more attainable goals, such as determining how to help your child and your entire family enjoy a happier, healthier life.

Double-Task, Don't Multitask

According to social psychology studies, we all believe we can multitask better than we actually can. Parents should quit multitasking and start double-tasking.

What's the distinction between the two? Multi-tasking is described as doing two or more linked tasks that require the same effort. Split attention, such as writing a post while also checking your phone when it rings, can cause you to take longer to complete the things on your list due to the time spent shifting attention and orienting to each activity.

Returning phone calls while walking the dog, driving while listening to an audiobook, eating lunch outside in a park, or walking while working on a trendy new treadmill workstation are all examples of double-tasking.

Consider it "task-enhancing," which entails mixing a pleasurable activity with something neutral or less pleasurable, such as watching an interesting movie or listening to your favorite music while cleaning dishes or folding laundry.

Emotional States Should Be Recognized and Regarded

Those close to autistic children's parents typically portray them as martyrs or heroes. It puts the parent under pressure to ensure their child never feels "bad" or develops socially inappropriate feelings.

Children are a handful even when they are the most beautiful individuals on earth. Even the most dedicated parent can be overtaken by the added burden of leading a child with autism who has difficulties expressing feelings in a non-harmful way. As a result, it is vital to accept anger, frustration, hurt, and loss when they occur.

While it is vital to care for and protect a child with autism, the parent's needs, personalities, emotions, and health must also be considered.

Allow for Extra Preparation Time

When things get tough, especially for parents of autistic children, they frequently claim they don't care about their appearance. However, seasoned experts—caretakers, fathers, and mothers who have seen it firsthand—advise that this is a dangerous viewpoint. Before leaping from the bed and running into all the things that must be performed, take a moment to care for the person in the mirror. Dress to please yourself, give special attention to your grooming routine, and go into the day prepared for whatever comes your way.

Pay Attention to Areas You Desire Development

Find methods to enjoy everything beautiful in your life, and you'll be astonished at how much more you discover.

Make your child laugh several times before school. Feel grateful for your excellent health and the efficient operation of all your body's unique systems. Thank your partner for making your coffee or taking out the garbage.

While you're at it, attempt to identify the constant chatter in your thoughts. Everyone has that little narrator who chatters non-stop all day. It is possible to modify the tone of your voice to a gentler one to avoid negativity.

Find Uplifters

Uplifters are those who encourage and support others. Parents with autistic children with a different worldview often find themselves surrounded by individuals who unwittingly discourage or cause them to acquire bad emotions. While they are usually loved ones, they should not be the only source of social engagement. Instead, make time to interact with adults who can bring helpful thoughts and emotions to the conversation. Make new friends that introduce you to new ideas and provide an adult-only outlet. Many parents miss the fact that parents must express and develop their identities outside of their jobs as parents.

Connect with Nature

There are vitamins and nutrients that human beings get from the sun, so spending time outdoors is something you should try to do at least a few times each week. Spend 30 minutes in your backyard and relax while getting some fresh air. Get away from the kids and go hiking, swim alone in the pool, or enjoy a picnic in your favorite park. Simply step outside and take in the sun's rays and the fresh air. People who spend time in green spaces such as local parks or other natural settings have better mental health and are more psychologically lively than those who do not.

Some Final Thoughts

Each day may feel like combat when you're fighting everybody, from your health insurer to your relatives who are not certain if your kid has autism or not and educators not going through with the individualized education program.

While a few fights may last a long time, you will realize others are not worth the trouble. Perhaps it's hesitating to discuss autism with a friend who isn't attempting to understand. Perhaps it's giving up on arguing with the child about cutting their hair because of their sensory impairments and allowing it to grow. Whatever it could be, consider whether it is worth all the effort and whether taking a step backward will bring some comfort into your life.

As a parent caring for a child with ASD, allowing yourself some grace periods is an essential but often overlooked aspect of self-care. It's common to feel the familiar guilt of not doing everything as a caregiver. There is probably much more you don't know or things you might have missed out on, and you criticize yourself for these things. You might feel bad, discouraged, or even burned out. However, in certain situations, lowering your aims, being compassionate with yourself, and celebrating even minor victories will go a long way toward self-preservation, knowing you did your best given the situation. Experts believe that the capacity to care for yourself and your child significantly increases when you pull yourself up.

CONCLUSION

All things considered; ASD caregivers endorse a wide range of responsibilities for the sake of their child's well-being. Due to the nature of their special needs, caring for someone with ASD can be draining, not just physically, but emotionally and psychologically as well. Between helping them with everyday tasks like getting dressed or bathing, taking them to see doctors, accompanying their learning, and much more, the job is far from easy. In reality, only a few people have the patience and resilience required to carry out this mission. But in the end, it's bound to be a rewarding experience.

As we've seen in this insightful book, caregivers must learn to balance their own needs and those of the person under their responsibility. Tending to all these duties can take a heavy toll on them, meaning they won't be able to provide the quality care all ASD sufferers need. This, in turn, can prompt sentiments of guilt, inadequacy, feeling like they can't handle it, and wanting to throw in the towel out of sheer frustration. Experiencing these emotions from time to time is normal, but it starts to become a warning sign that something is wrong when the caregiver feels they can no longer administer the care the child needs to thrive.

Throughout these pages, we've explored how important it is for ASD caregivers to be able to prioritize self-care for their own sake. Adopting a positive outlook on every situation can grant them the motivation to pursue the child's development and allow them to lead a normal life. This is achieved thanks to small daily rituals, such as finding ways to relieve stress, taking periodic breaks, and making time to do things that remind us to enjoy living our lives. Whenever things get particularly difficult, and the stress runs high, seeking help from a trusted outside source might be necessary. That's especially true for children who need constant supervision. Doing so gives the caregiver a chance to re-evaluate the situation, regroup, and refresh. Time away is also a useful remedy for regaining the strength to face new future challenges.

When all is said and done, self-care for caregivers is a necessity if you want to survive the rigors of the challenges ahead. But while dealing with the problems that come with ASD can feel like a burden, it's vital to recognize that the person you're caring for is not one. Everybody has something they need help with at different points throughout their lives, and people with ASD just need a little more love and attention.

There's a reason why the verbiage surrounding ASD has changed from things like "an autistic child" to "a child with autism" or "a child with ASD." We have to remember that, while it is a trait of such individuals, it isn't *the* defining trait. People with ASD can live long and happy lives, and you can be there right alongside them, laughing during the good times, crying during the sad ones, and being an integral part of the life of someone very special.

By applying all the tips and advice found in the guide, ASD caregivers will be able to better manage and preserve their mental health in the long run. With that, they'll succeed in providing the best level of care possible for their loved ones. Remember that this is a process that can take months, even years, so giving yourself ample time to adjust is primordial. And of course, if you feel you could benefit from talking to someone yourself, don't delay seeking help. In the end, it's in everyone's best interest!

REFERENCES

5 Self Care Tips for adults with autism. (2019, January 11). ABA Degree Programs; Applied Behavior Analysis Degree Programs. https://www.abadegreeprograms.net/lists/5-self-care-tips-for-adults-with-autism/

8 self-care ideas for parents of autistic children during the holidays. (2018, December 2). Applied Behavior Analysis Programs Guide. https://www.appliedbehavioranalysisprograms.com/lists/5-self-care-ideas-for-parents-of-autistic-children-during-the-holidays/

9 health benefits of music. (2017, July 24). Northshore.Org. https://www.northshore.org/healthy-you/9-health-benefits-of-music/

20 self-care ideas for caregivers. (2017, April 18). Little Mama Jama. http://littlemamajama.com/20-self-care-ideas-for-caregivers/

Al-Dujaili, A. H., & Al-Mossawy, D. A. J. (2017). Psychosocial burden among caregivers of children with autism spectrum disorder in Najaf province. Current Pediatric Research. https://www.currentpediatrics.com/articles/psychosocia

l-burden-among-caregivers-of-children-with-autism-spectrumdisorder-in-najaf-province.html

Alshahrani, M. S., & Algashmari, H. (2021). The moderating effect of financial stress and autism severity on development of depression among parents and caregivers of Autistic children in Taif, Saudi Arabia. Journal of Family Medicine and Primary Care, 10(3), 1227–1233. https://doi.org/10.4103/jfmpc.jfmpc_2203_20

Amy Morin, L. (2019, July 17). Best mental health apps. Verywell Mind. https://www.verywellmind.com/best-mental-health-apps-4692902

Britton, R. (n.d.). Self-care tips for parents with autistic children. Clinical-Partners.Co.Uk. https://www.clinical-partners.co.uk/insights-and-news/family-issues/item/self-care-tips-for-parents-with-autistic-children

CDC. (2022, March 31). What is Autism Spectrum Disorder? Centers for Disease Control and Prevention. https://www.cdc.gov/ncbddd/autism/facts.html

Dada-Olley, L. (2021, June 28). Caregiver's chronicles: Self-care is how I care. Psych Central. https://psychcentral.com/health/self-care-essential-to-caregivers

Friesen, K. A., Weiss, J. A., Howe, S. J., Kerns, C. M., & McMorris, C. A. (2022). Mental health and resilient coping in caregivers of autistic individuals during the COVID-19 pandemic: Findings from the families facing COVID study. Journal of Autism and Developmental Disorders, 52(7), 3027–3037. https://doi.org/10.1007/s10803-021-05177-4

Hart, T. H. (2022, May 16). Caregiver self-care guide: 10 ways parents of a child with autism can make space for themselves. The Elemy Learning Studio. https://www.elemy.com/studio/autism-family-guide/caregiver-self-care/

Helping your child with autism thrive - HelpGuide.Org. (n.d.). https://www.helpguide.org/articles/autism-learning-disabilities/helping-your-child-with-autism-thrive.htm

How parents and caregivers of kids with autism cope with stress. (2021, May 20). LEARN Behavioral. https://learnbehavioral.com/blog/how-parents-and-caregivers-of-kids-with-autism-cope-with-stress

Keighery, M. (2017, December 18). Taking care of yourself, taking care of your child with Autism. WayAhead; WayAhead - Mental Health Association NSW. https://wayahead.org.au/taking-care-of-yourself-taking-care-of-your-child-with-autism/

Koutsimani, P., Montgomery, A., & Georganta, K. (2019). The relationship between burnout, depression, and anxiety: A systematic review and meta-analysis. Frontiers in Psychology, 10, 284. https://doi.org/10.3389/fpsyg.2019.00284

Lai, W. W., & Oei, T. P. S. (2014). Coping in parents and caregivers of children with autism spectrum disorders (ASD): A review. Review-Journal of Autism and Developmental Disorders, 1(3), 207–224. https://doi.org/10.1007/s40489-014-0021-x

Leo Newhouse, L. (2021, March 1). Is crying good for you? Harvard Health. https://www.health.harvard.edu/blog/is-crying-good-for-you-2021030122020

Marcin, A. (2017, February 27). Are 5-minute daily workout routines really beneficial? Healthline. https://www.healthline.com/health/5-minute-daily-workout-routines-really-beneficial

Meditation: A simple, fast way to reduce stress. (2022, April 29). Mayo Clinic. https://www.mayoclinic.org/tests-procedures/meditation/in-depth/meditation/art-20045858

Mental health benefits of journaling. (n.d.). WebMD. https://www.webmd.com/mental-health/mental-health-benefits-of-journaling

Mierow, L. (2021). Tips for parenting A child with autism: Help you effectively manage everyday situations: Types of autism spectrum disorder. Independently Published.

Nurturing ourselves: 10 self-care tips for autism parents. (2021, May 14). RDIconnect | Parent and Professional Training; RDIconnect. https://www.rdiconnect.com/nurturing-ourselves-10-self-care-tips-for-autism-parents/

Papera, K. (2020, March 10). Self-care for autism parents and caregivers —. Behavior Frontiers. https://www.behaviorfrontiers.com/blog/self-care-for-parents-and-caregivers

Parenting autistic children, the challenges, and rewards. (2016, November 16). Autism 360 Support. https://www.autism360support.com/parenting-autism/

Psychological benefits of routines. (n.d.). WebMD. https://www.webmd.com/mental-health/psychological-benefits-of-routine

Reconciliation of work and family life - statistics. (n.d.). Europa.Eu. https://ec.europa.eu/eurostat/statistics-explained/index.php?title=Reconciliation_of_work_and_family_life_-_statistics

Scott, E. (2018, February 5). The benefits of meditation for stress management. Verywell Mind. https://www.verywellmind.com/meditation-4157199

Self-care & stress management tips for parents of children with autism and special needs. (2021, July 28). Behavioral Innovations - ABA Therapy for Kids with Autism. https://behavioral-innovations.com/blog/self-care-stress-management-tips/

Self-care for Adults who Care for Children with Autism. (n.d.). Mayinstitute.Org. https://www.mayinstitute.org/news/acl/asd-and-dd-adult-focused/self-care-for-adults-who-care-for-children-with-autism/

Shazeen Ahmad, M. A. (2020, November 30). Coping strategies for autism caregivers. Autism Parenting Magazine. https://www.autismparentingmagazine.com/autism-caregivers-coping-strategies/

Smith, K., & LPC. (2018, December 19). Coping with stress while caring for a child with autism. Psycom.Net - Mental Health Treatment Resource Since 1996; Psycom.net. https://www.psycom.net/coping-with-stress-while-caring-for-a-child-with-autism/

Special Learning House. (2022, March 4). 5 minute self-care ideas for autism caregivers (33 awesome ideas).

Special Learning House.
https://www.speciallearninghouse.com/5-minute-self-care-ideas/

Stebbins, L. F., & M Ed M L I. (n.d.). Autism parents: How do you rate on self-care? Stageslearning.Com https://blog.stageslearning.com/blog/autism-parents-self-care

Stress relievers: Tips to tame stress. (2021, March 18). Mayo Clinic. https://www.mayoclinic.org/healthy-lifestyle/stress-management/in-depth/stress-relievers/art-20047257

The Mom Kind. (2021, May 14). 7 self-care tips for parents of special needs children. The Mom Kind • Autism Parenting Advice • Neurodiverse Parenting Resourse; The Mom Kind 501(c)(3). https://themomkind.com/7-self-care-tips-for-parents-of-special-needs-children/

Upham, B., & Mackenzie, S. (n.d.). Self-care for autism caregivers. EverydayHealth.Com. https://www.everydayhealth.com/autism/how-to-care-for-yourself-when-you-re-caring-for-someone-with-autism/

Ventola, P., Lei, J., Paisley, C., Lebowitz, E., & Silverman, W. (2017). Parenting a child with ASD: Comparison of parenting style between ASD, anxiety, and typical development. Journal of Autism and Developmental Disorders, 47(9), 2873–2884. https://doi.org/10.1007/s10803-017-3210-5

Weil, A. T. (2003). Taking care of yourself: Strategies for eating well, staying fit and living in balance. ABC Audio.

What does too much screen time do to children's brains? (2019, August 8). NewYork-Presbyterian. https://healthmatters.nyp.org/what-does-too-much-screen-time-do-to-childrens-brains/

Wigginton, P. (2020, June 20). The importance of self-care for the ASD caregiver. Autism Parenting Magazine. https://www.autismparentingmagazine.com/self-care-for-the-asd-caregiver/